ABANDONED TOPEKA

PSYCHIATRIC CAPITAL OF THE WORLD

EMILY COWAN

AMERICA THROUGH TIME®
ADDING COLOR TO AMERICAN HISTORY

This book is dedicated to my mother, my biggest supporter and cheerleader. Mom, I would not be the person I am or as successful today without your continuous support and allowing me the freedom to make mistakes, explore, and try new things. I love you.

America Through Time is an imprint of Fonthill Media LLC
www.through-time.com
office@through-time.com

Published by Arcadia Publishing by arrangement with Fonthill Media LLC
For all general information, please contact Arcadia Publishing:
Telephone: 843-853-2070
Fax: 843-853-0044
E-mail: sales@arcadiapublishing.com
For customer service and orders:
Toll-Free 1-888-313-2665

www.arcadiapublishing.com

First published 2022

ISBN 978-1-63499-374-6

Typeset in Trade Gothic 10pt on 15pt
Printed and bound in England

CONTENTS

ABOUT THE AUTHOR

EMILY COWAN was born and raised in Kansas until she was ten, living just twenty minutes outside of the capital city. She spent plenty of time in Topeka hanging out with family, shopping, and going out to do things. She moved to Oklahoma but has stayed in touch with her roots over the years, going back numerous times in a year. In January of 2020, she was brought onto the Abandoned Oklahoma team, where she fell in love with photojournalism and history. She knew that kickstarting Abandoned Kansas was without a doubt a goal she wanted to achieve sooner rather than later. What better place to start than back to Topeka to learn all about the places she hadn't noticed when she was younger.

INTRODUCTION

While I no longer live in Topeka, the Sunflower State is and always will be the place I call home. I lived in the Topeka area until I was ten, so my knowledge of the history of the city's buildings wasn't abundant. As I got older, I realized there were a lot of things that high school history classes didn't teach me about the state I was currently living in. This curiosity followed me back to Topeka on my monthly trips home. I would pass by what seemed to be a score of abandoned buildings scattered through the Golden City. Come with me to some of my favorite locations in the "Psychiatric Capital of the World" and hopefully learn a thing or two along the way!

1

MENNINGER CLINIC

Security Benefit Association

Before there was Menninger's, there were just eleven men on a winter day in December 1891 pooling together a dollar each to create a security fund for those of minuscule wealth. The Knights and Ladies of Security was officially established on February 22, 1892, with the organized assistance of Dr. H. A. Warner and George H. Flintham. The fraternal society was inclusive of women, the poor, children, and the elderly, providing insurance and social security to protect from the uncertainties of life. The organization spread like wildfire; by 1895, they had memberships in the thousands and around 328 local councils in Kansas and surrounding states.

The years of 1916-17 were big for the organization, as this was when the foundation for their campus would be established. Knights and Ladies of Security were each asked to contribute five cents to go towards the construction of the mutual cooperative farm, home, and hospital. Funds would later be used for a school and hotel on the grounds. The hospital became one of the best in the city and the home for the elderly was created around a model farm. In later years, an orphanage was built along with the school to care for children whose parents were members of Knights and Ladies of Security and had passed away. All of these benefits were offered to members for just a nickel a month. By 1919, the organization had grown substantially and merged with another company to become the Security Benefit Association.

The new version of the hospital was constructed of limestone and brick and three stories high with a 140-foot clock tower in the center. Being added to the grounds in 1924 as one central building that would cost around $250,000 initially. Deemed a replica of Independence Hall in Philadelphia, the hospital opened officially in 1925, but it wasn't long before the SBA determined that they would need a bigger facility.

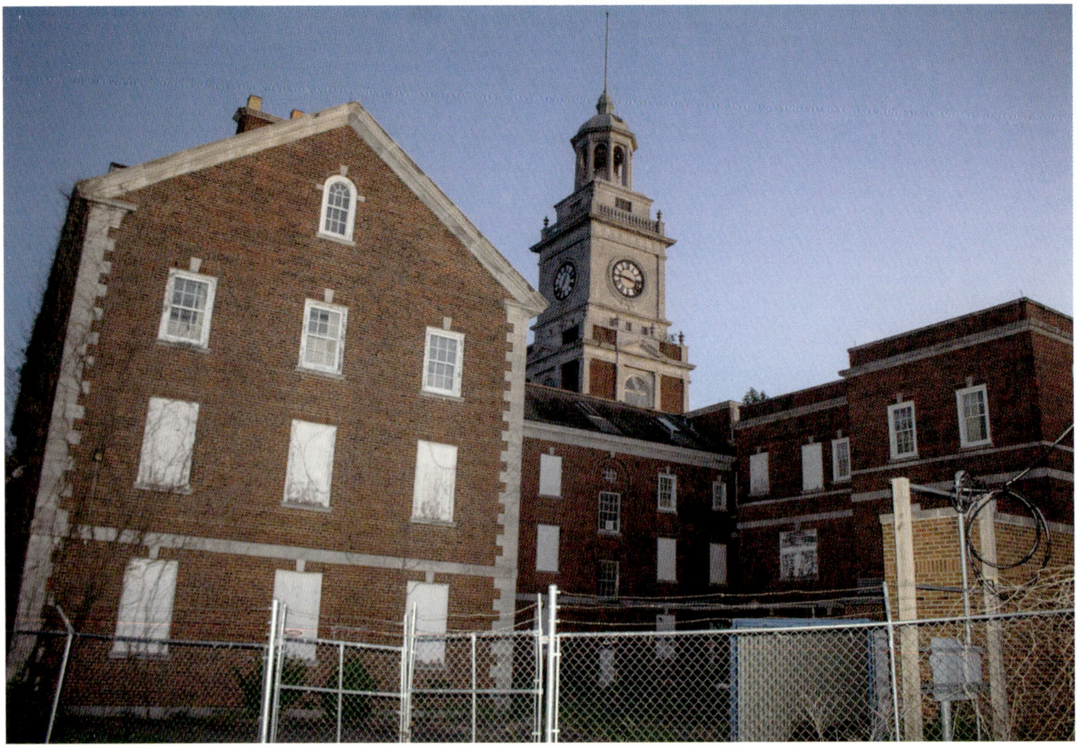

Menningers Clocktower at Dusk.

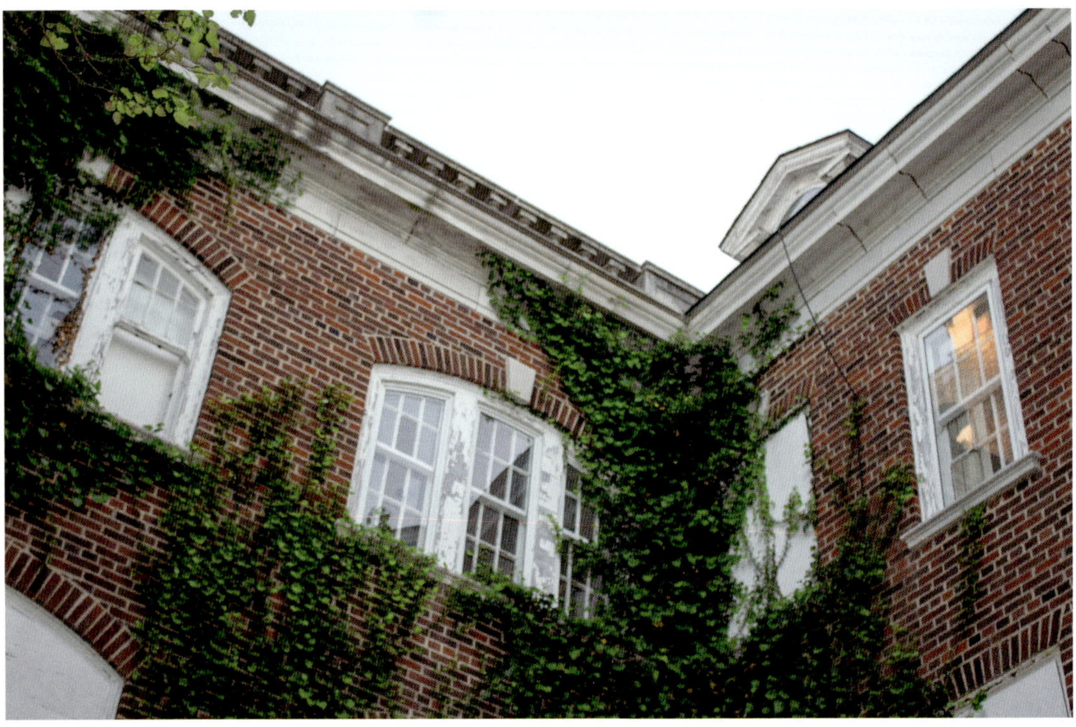

Vines growing up the north wall.

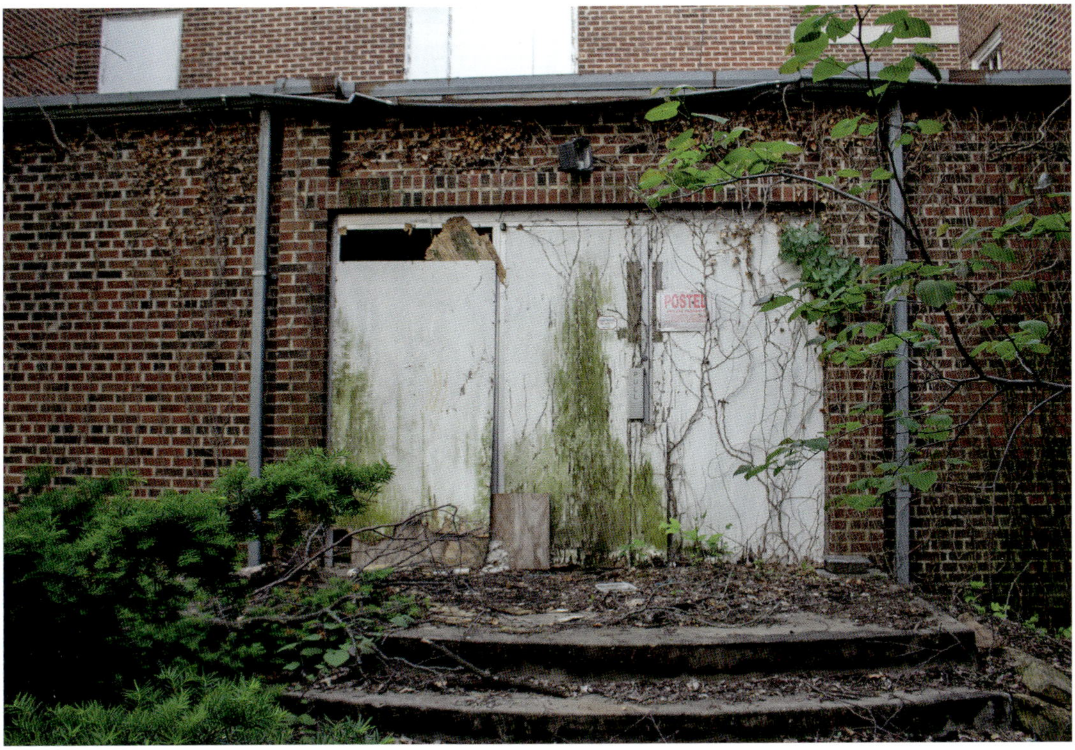

Boarded-up entrance.

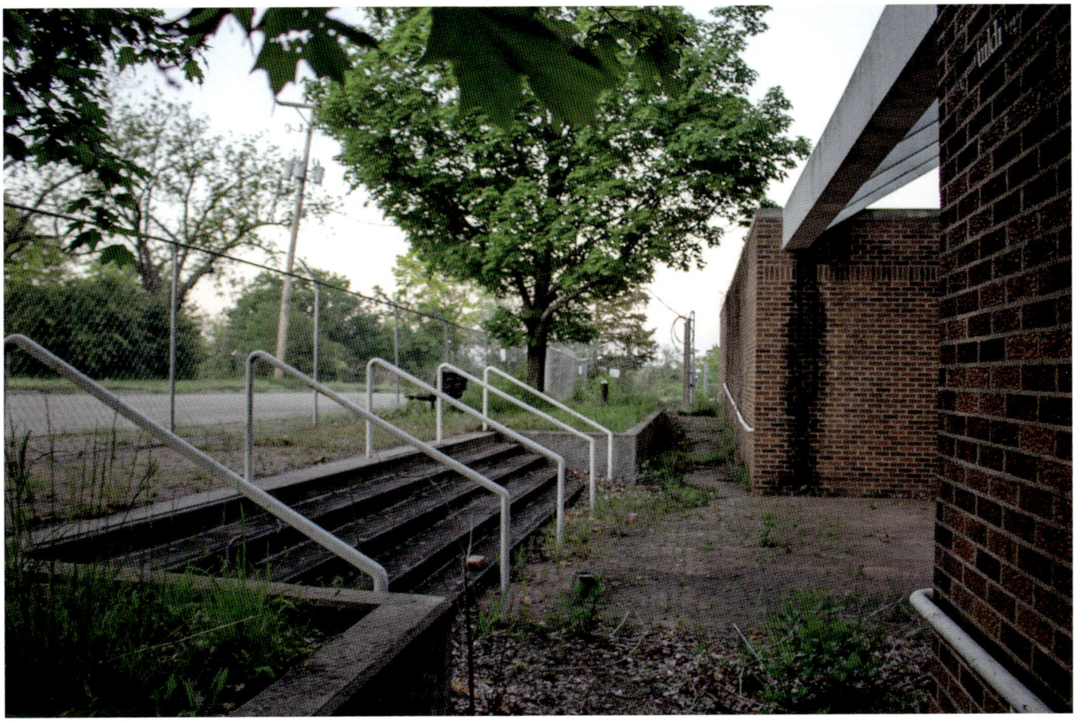

Stairs leading to the north entrance.

The largest building project since the Hotel Jayhawk was underway on Martin's Hill in the fall of 1928. The enlargement would cost no less than $300,000 to complete the two identical wings. They would be added on to each end, connecting them to the central building and creating space for 200 more beds. New kitchen facilities and a nurses' dining room, in addition to fifteen clinic rooms, two laboratories, a physical therapy room, and five operating rooms were also included. After allegedly no admissions since 1941, the Security Benefit Association shifted its focus and closed down the Security Benefit Home and Hospital in 1954.

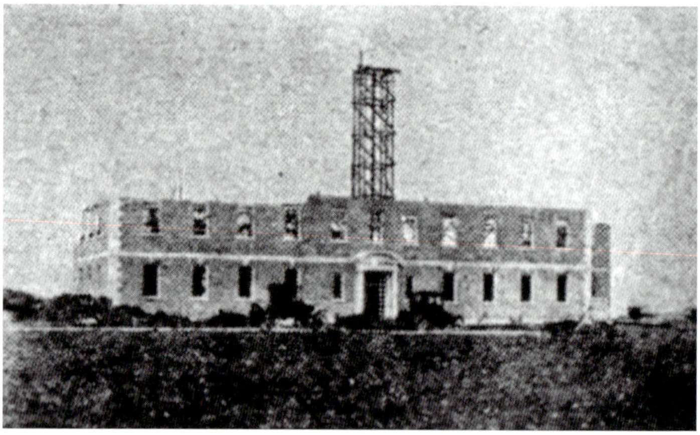

Central Building under construction *ca.* 1924.

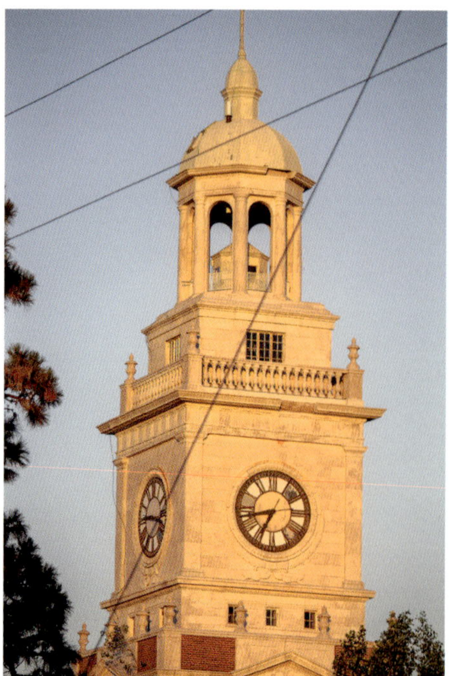

Sun beaming off the vacant clocktower.

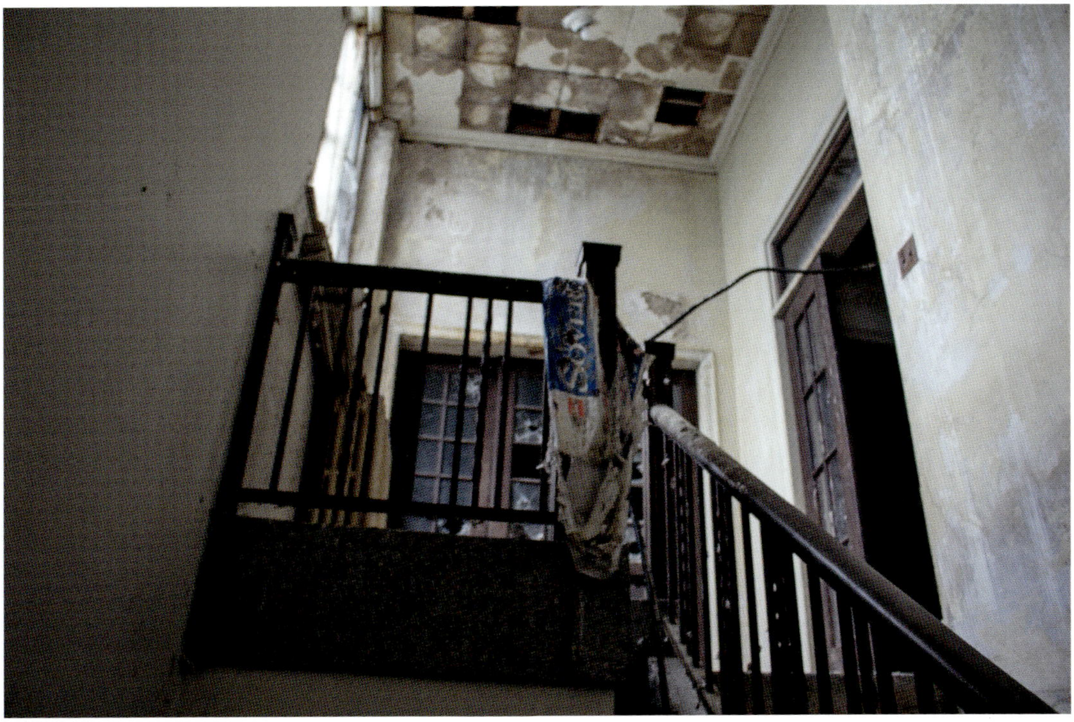

Stairs leading up to the clocktower.

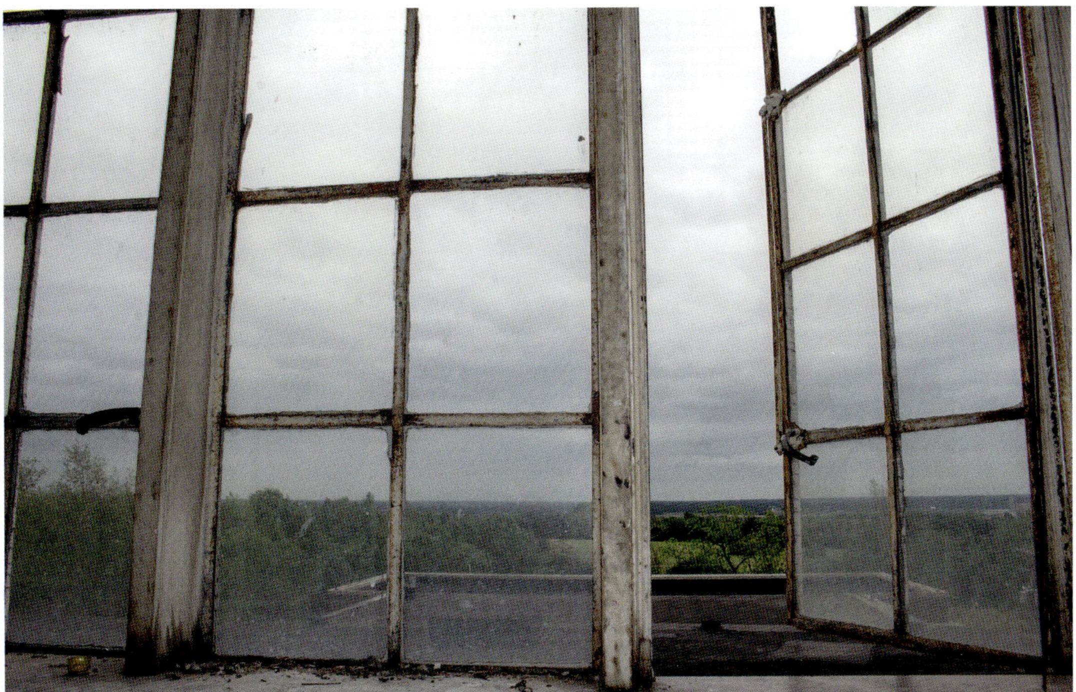

View out of the upper floor window facing north.

Menninger Sanitarium (East Campus)

Menninger might as well be a household name throughout Topeka, as there isn't a family in town that doesn't know of the Menninger's. The Menninger Clinic was started by father and son duo, Dr. Charles and Dr. Karl Menninger, in 1925, after fascination in the psychiatric industry overcame them. The first building on what became known as the East Campus of Menninger's Sanitarium was a farmhouse that sat on twenty acres in Topeka, fit with twelve beds.

Eventually, the Sanitarium grew to a flourishing campus, including Topeka Institute for Psychoanalysis, Clinic Building, two research buildings, two libraries, multiple educational buildings, C. F. Menninger Memorial Hospital, Child Psychiatric services, nurses housing, and lodges. Southard School for children was located at East Campus and was one of the first institutions specifically for children with mental health disabilities, taking on a new way of treating the mentally ill and paving the way for a restructuring of treatment throughout America.

As the Menninger's work and campus continued to grow, so did the need for funding. Thus, the Menninger's Foundation was born in 1941 as a registered 501(c)(3) non-profit organization. This allowed for more funds to be moved around in the operation and expansion of buildings and programs to be brought in. The Menninger School of Psychiatry was one of those programs. Established in 1946, it became one of the largest psychiatric training centers in the country. This was the start to one of the biggest and most advanced psychiatric education revolutions of the post-WWII era. It became the main hub for students training in psychology and mental health disorders. The "new" therapies integrated into the program involved those of medical, developmental, family, and emotional/physical/social needs to help improve patients. This campus treated thousands of patients and taught thousands of student psychoanalysts up until a new and larger campus was needed.

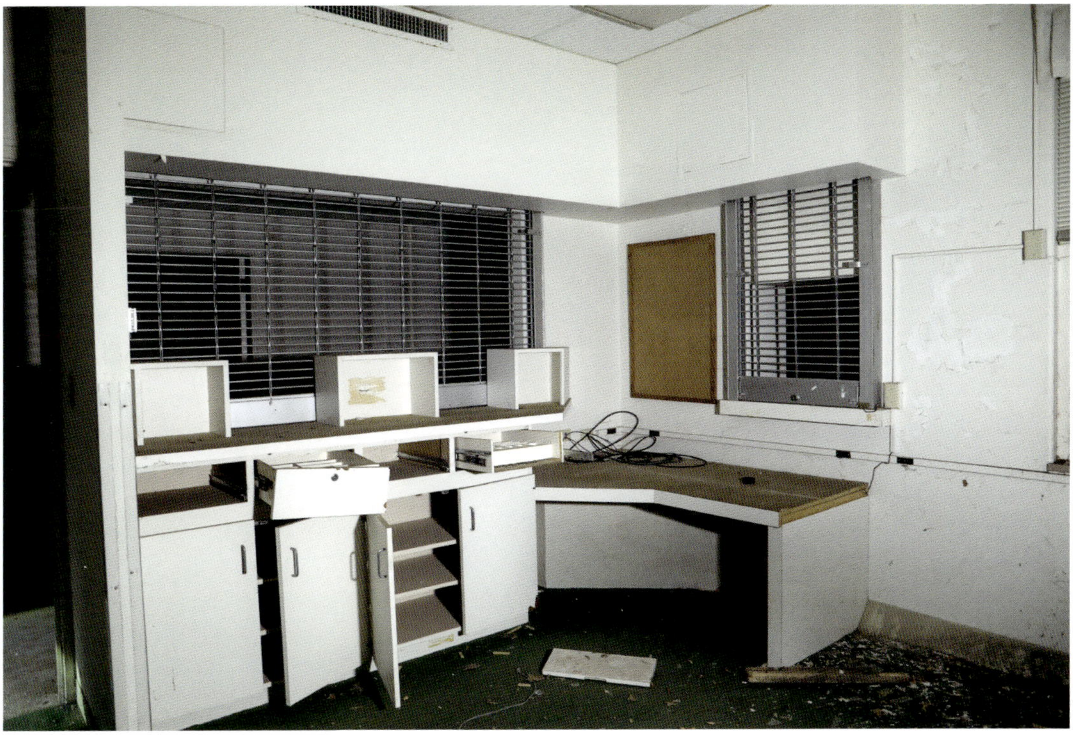

Closed right now, please see the front desk for help.

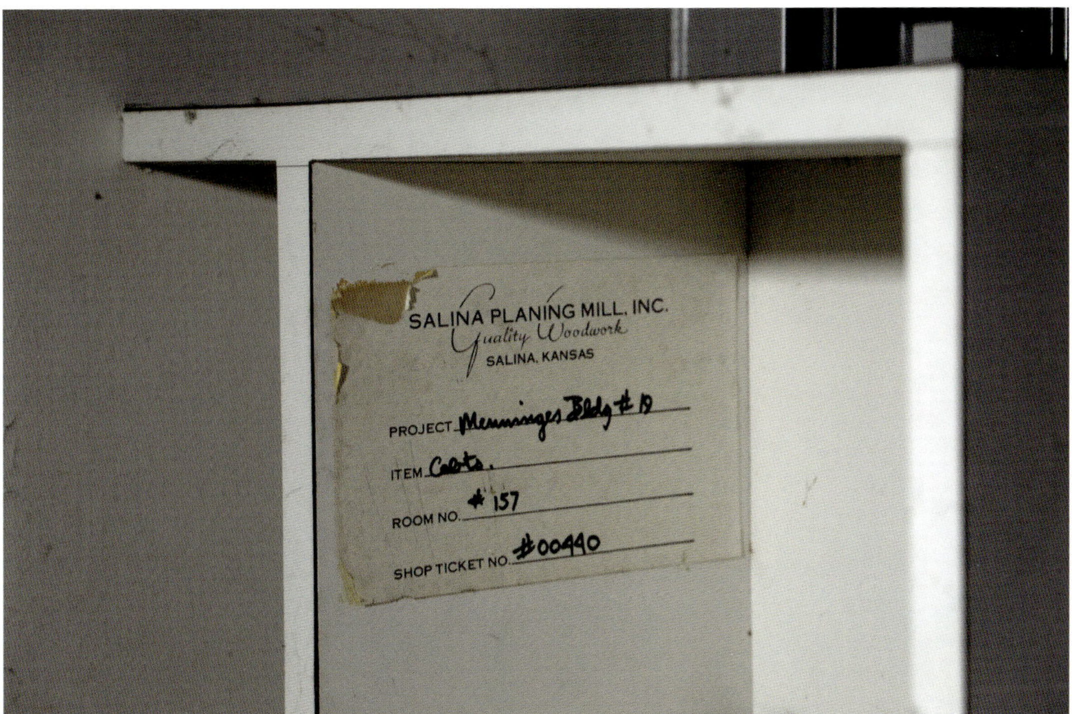

Menningers Building #19.

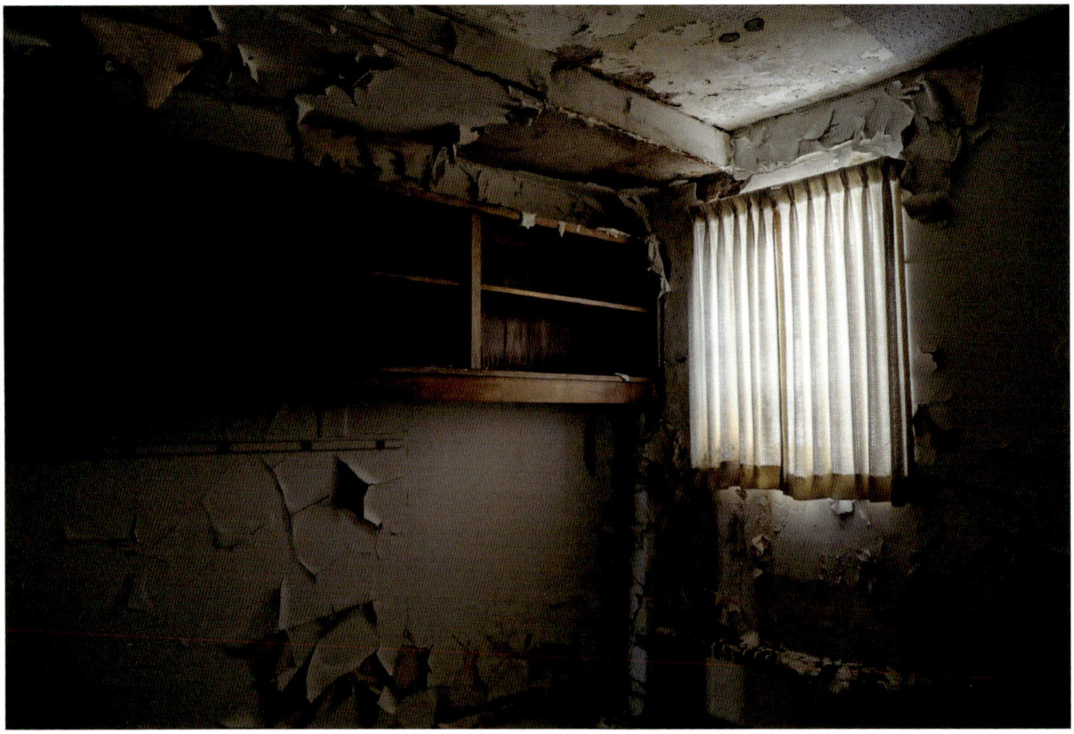

Curtains closed, please.

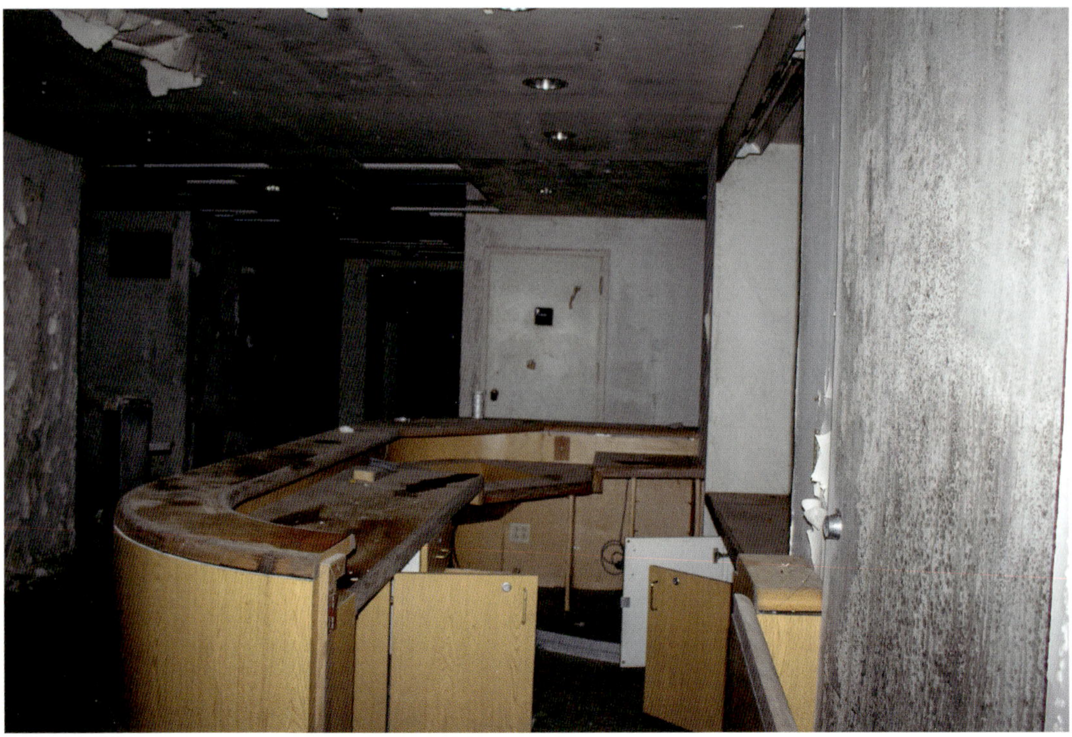

Front desk of Tower Building.

Menninger Clinic (West Campus)

Sitting lifelessly for five years, the complex of buildings that used to be Security Benefit Home and Hospital was bought up by the growing Menninger's Foundation in 1959. This would become West Campus, which already had fifteen buildings that just needed a little modernization and renovating. This brought the total number of buildings to thirty-nine, equaling 430 acres, with a staff of around 1,000 and a $17,000,000 annual budget. After assessing the Menninger Foundations' buildings and programs in 1975, it was determined that consolidating the two campuses clinics, educational, and research buildings into one campus would be financially smart and beneficial for the foundation. The East Campus had buildings over fifty years old, and it was decided that further developing and consolidating to the West Campus would be the smartest move. On May 1, 1980, groundbreaking for the $35 million project was underway and the development of Menninger's West Campus would soon become the hub of the thriving psychiatric industry in Topeka.

The new buildings would be a place for people who treat, who are treated, who teach, who learn and who generate new knowledge with their research.

> The thing that impresses me about Menninger's is that they carry the work they do on their patients out into the community—they were doing this before anyone else. They also have developed unique screening processes for servicemen and potential psychiatrists. I don't know of any other groups that have done the sort of thing they have.
>
> Dr. Geoffrey Osier, member of the American Board of Psychiatry and Neurology

The main building (former SBA Hospital Building) was truthfully the center of the West Campus, the eye-catcher, a staple piece in the Topeka skyline. The beauty and detail of the clocktower that sits in the center is something that all Topekans recognize to this day. The power plant was used to power the campus and included a laundry unit within it. A pool was located in between the power plant and Building D, which was a four-story brick, steel, and concrete building consisting of twenty-eight rooms. In addition, others on the West Campus included Building A, a three-story brick building consisting of twenty-four rooms, equipped with a kitchen and cafeteria. Buildings B & C were three-stories tall with B having twenty-eight rooms. Building E was fitted with eight apartments for executive personnel and fifty rooms, and Building G was of brick and wood. The reservoir held two-and-a-half million gallons for emergencies.

The Menninger Foundation changed the way psychiatric practices were done all over the United States and was for decades one of the top facilities in the Midwest.

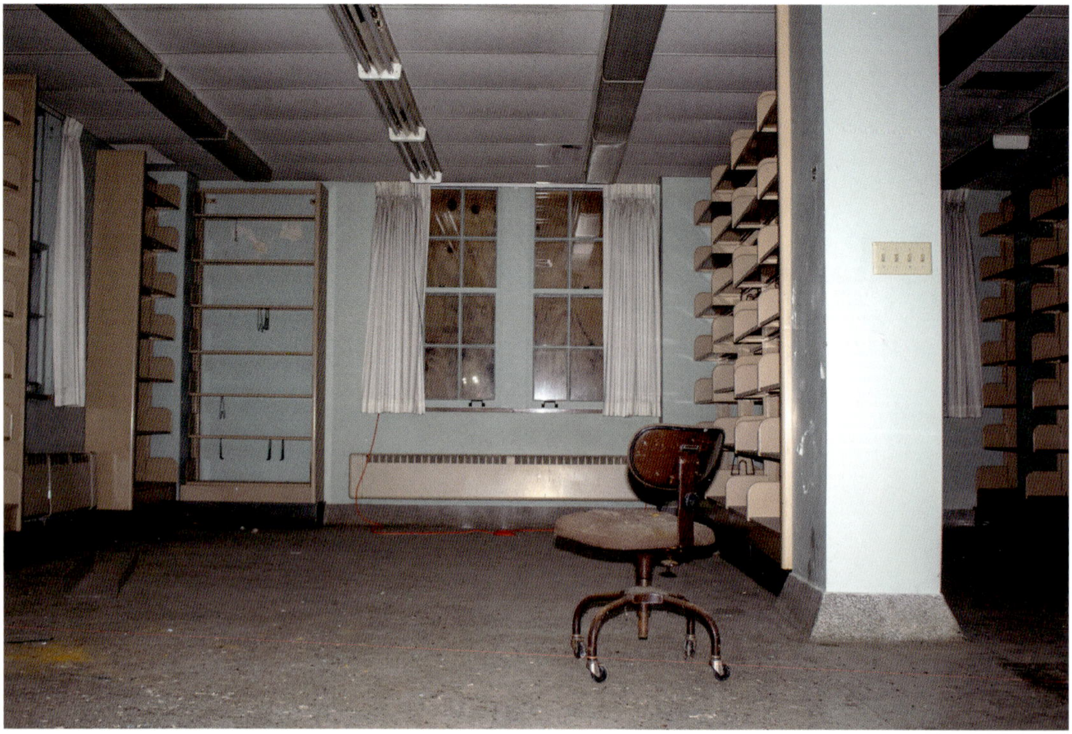

Lonely chair in the files room.

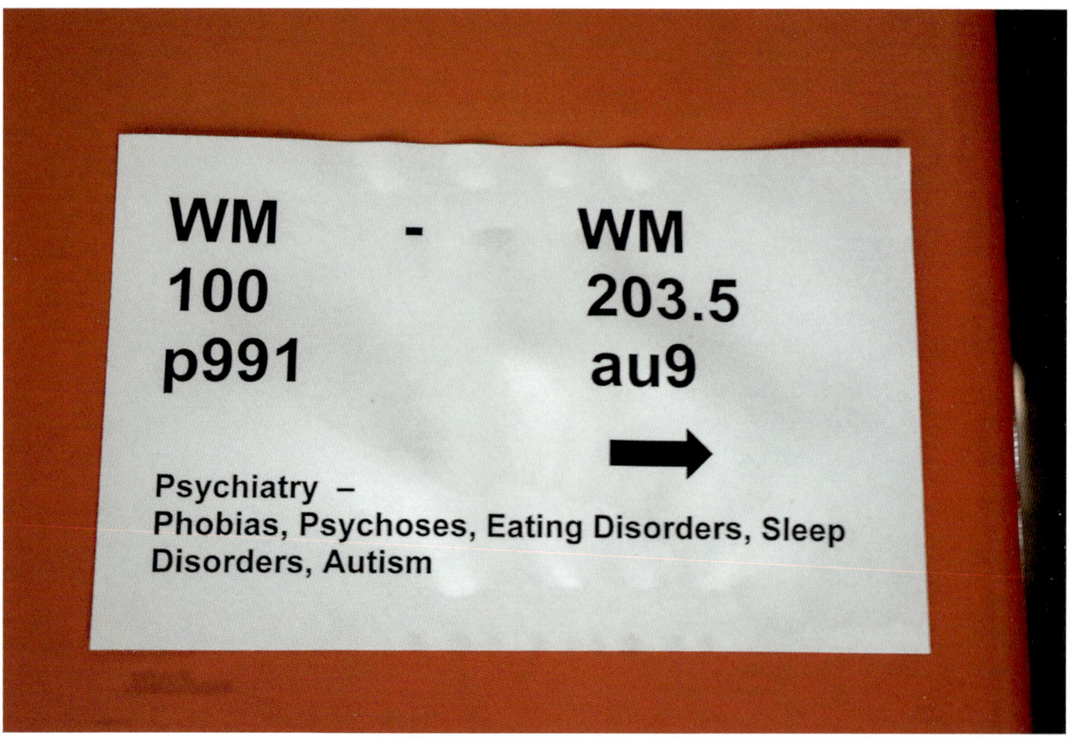

Files on phobias, psychoses, eating disorders, sleep disorders, and autism on this shelf.

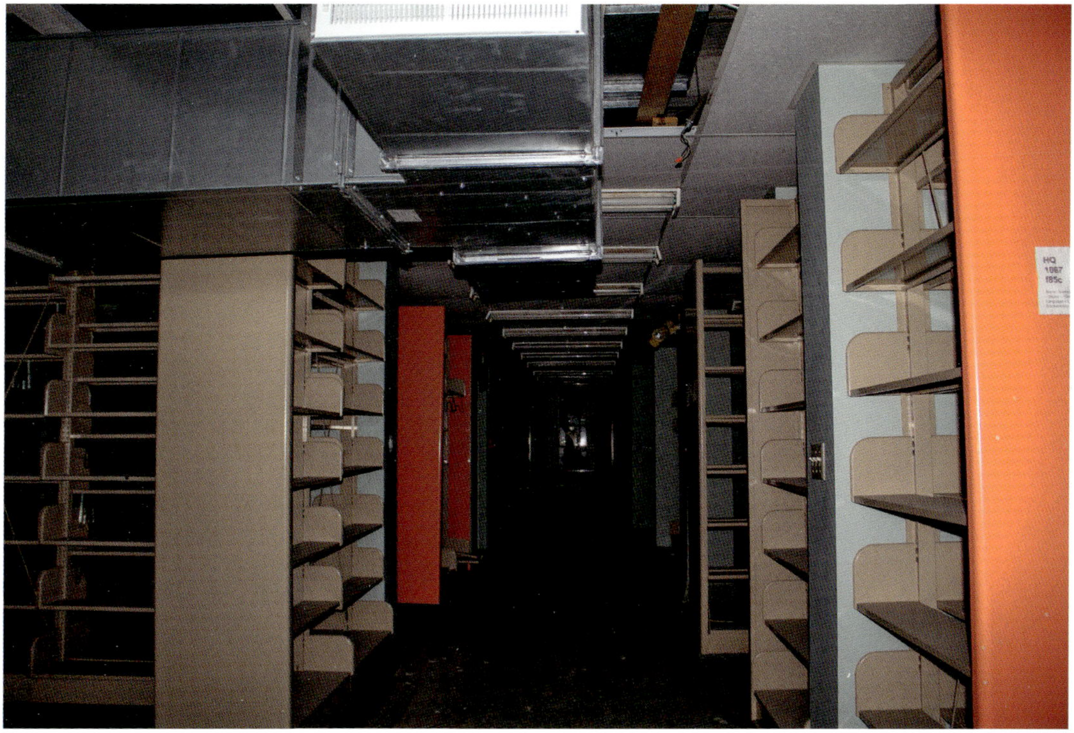

Rows and rows of shelves for files.

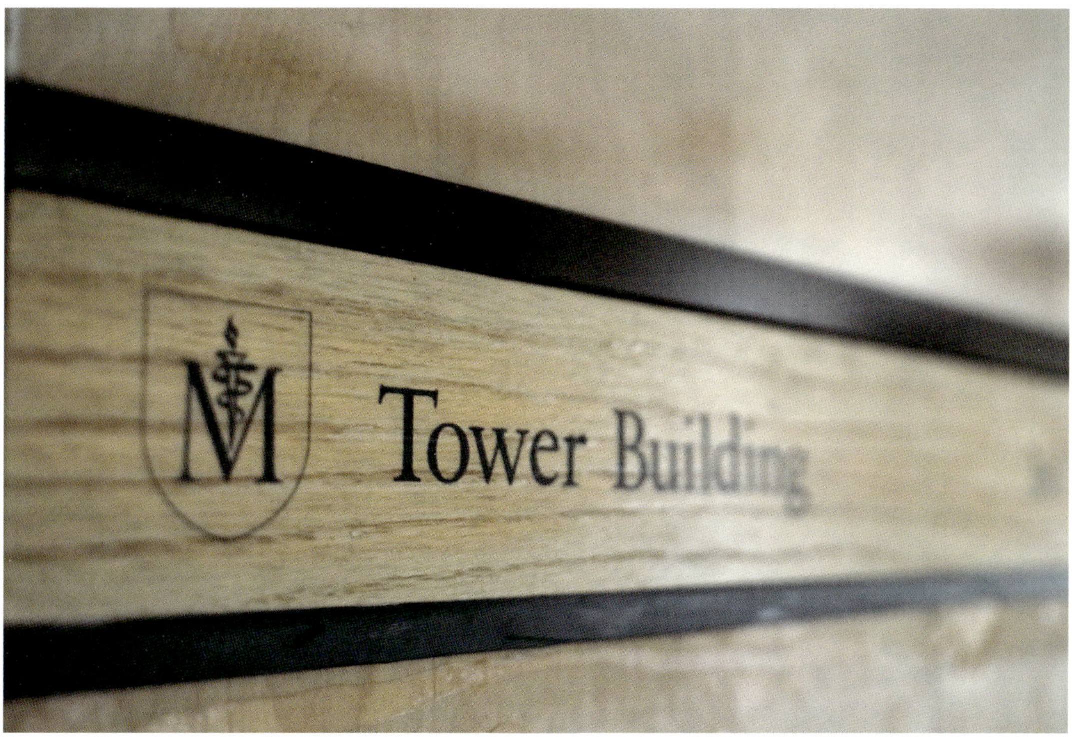

Tower Building first floor.

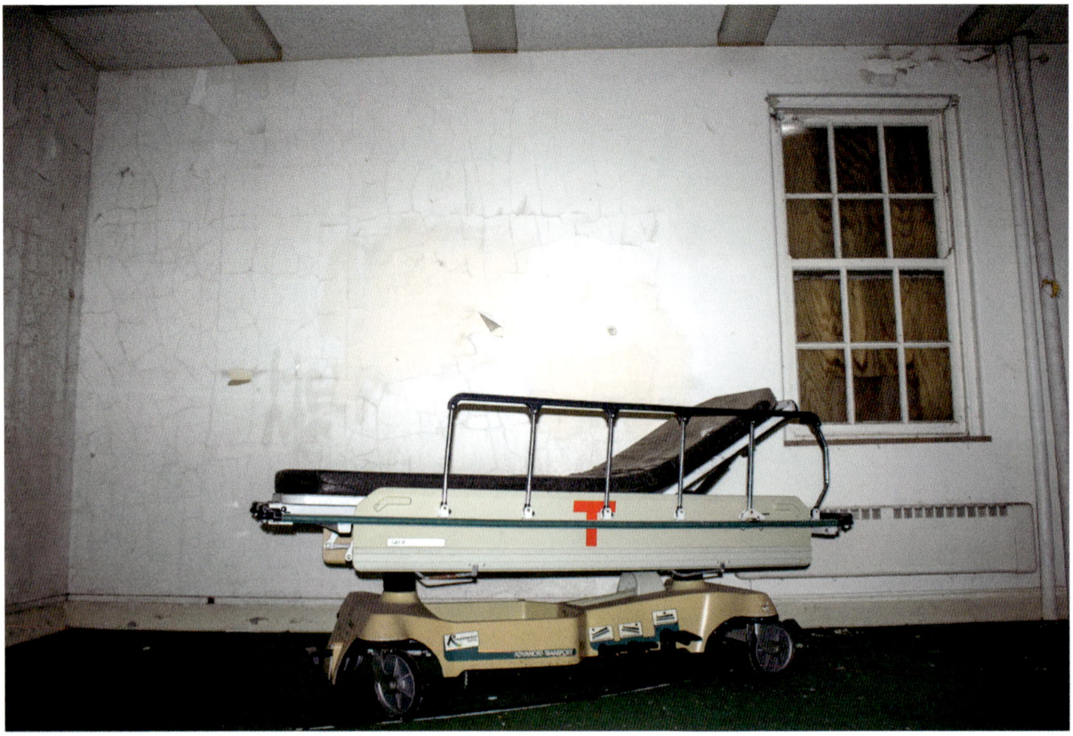

Last hospital bed.

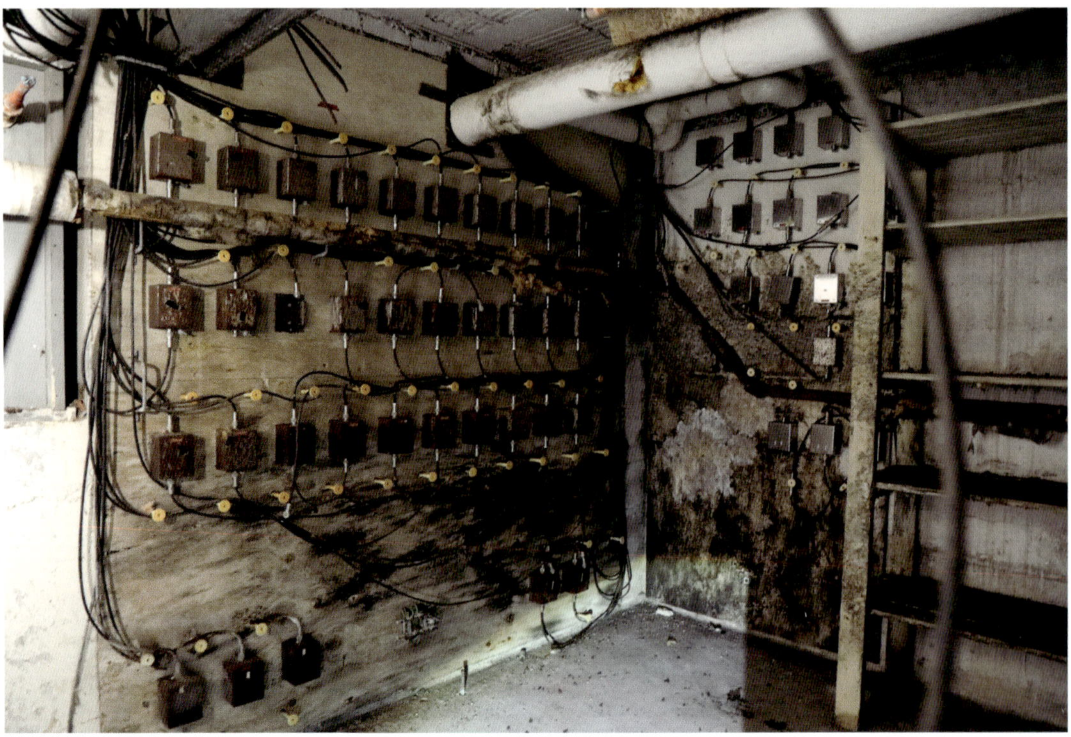

Basement room.

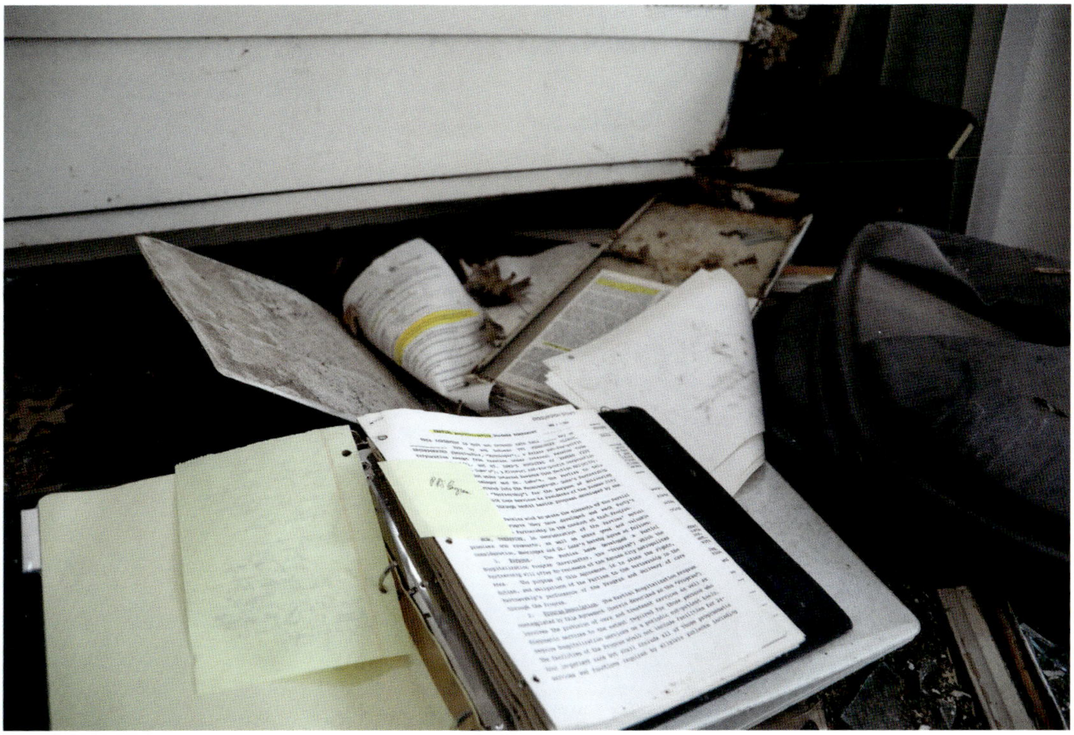

Partial Hospitalization Program Agreement binder.

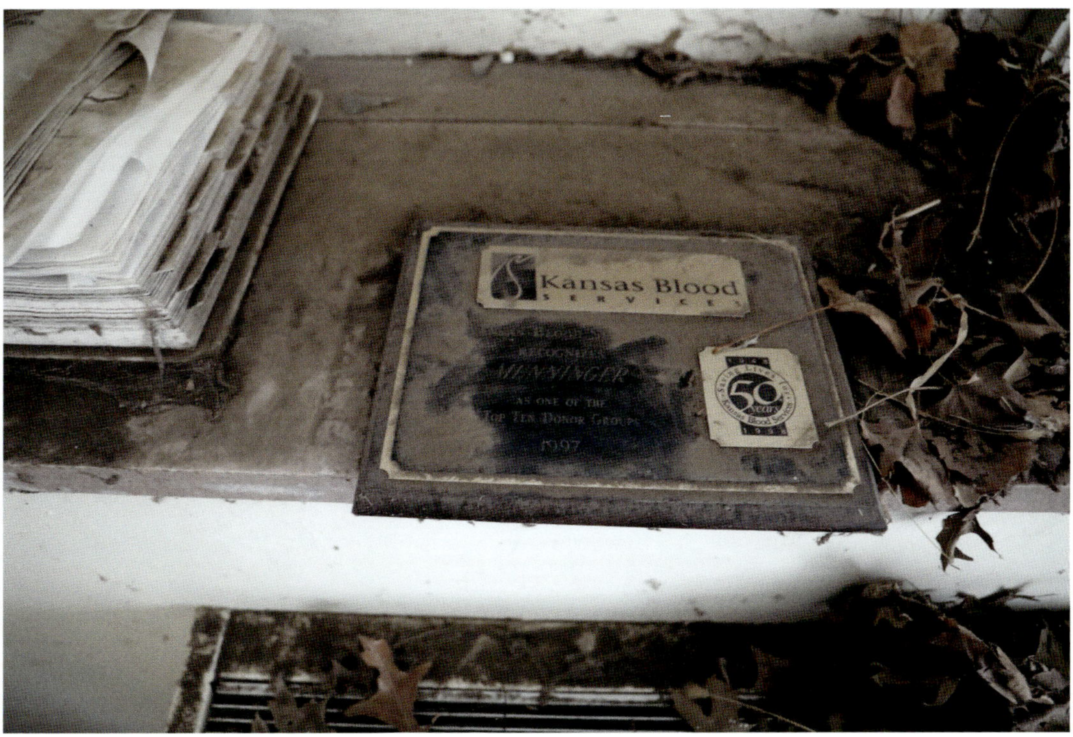

"Kansas Blood Services recognizes Menninger as one of the top ten donor groups 1997."

Research, education, and new and improved treatment of mental health issues were always the main focus of the operation. When the Menninger's Sanitarium was first brought to Topeka, the Founders and patients were not welcomed by Topekans. But after years of public outreach and education, the family managed to change how a lot of the community viewed and interacted with patients with mental disorders.

Frozen in Time

In the late 90s and early 2000s the Menninger Foundation started to experience financial stress as the treatment of patients changed and so did the facility's needs. Long-term patients that needed to be housed full time in its dormitories became less and less, which meant running the giant campus became more and more expensive. Health insurance coverage for mental health had changed and many plans no longer covered the treatment patients needed to receive, creating a further issue. September 27, 2000, Menninger's made its official announcement that it would be leaving not only Topeka but Kansas altogether, after more than seventy-five years in the Sunflower State. President Walt Menninger, son of William Menninger, had signed a letter of intent to work with Baylor College of Medicine and Methodist Health Care System to form an alliance in Houston, Texas. The move was to ensure the future of Menninger's would be secured, even if that meant leaving their roots behind.

Over the next three years, the clinic worked to move operations down south and figure outpatient situations. On May 31, 2003, the last twenty-nine patients boarded a jet to Houston, leaving Topeka the "Psychiatric Capital of the World" no more. Only eight psychiatrists were still staffed with the clinic versus the almost eighty that worked there just a few decades earlier. After the move, 3,400 boxes of Menningers archives were gifted to the Kansas State Historical Society, ensuring its history in Topeka would not be forgotten. They also donated 76 acres of land to the Kansas Department of Wildlife to become the Kaw River State Park.

Menninger's Hill underwent a different kind of cleansing starting in June 2008 when demolition crews stepped in to start the takedown of around fifteen old Menninger's buildings. The first to come down was the woodworking shop that was used as a patient care activity building. Saint Francis Health Center of Topeka had plans to develop the property, but after the 2008 recession, SCL Health transferred ownership of their Saint Francis Hospital to the University of Kansas health system. The deal outlined that the Sisters of Charity at Leavenworth could retain the Menninger Hill property.

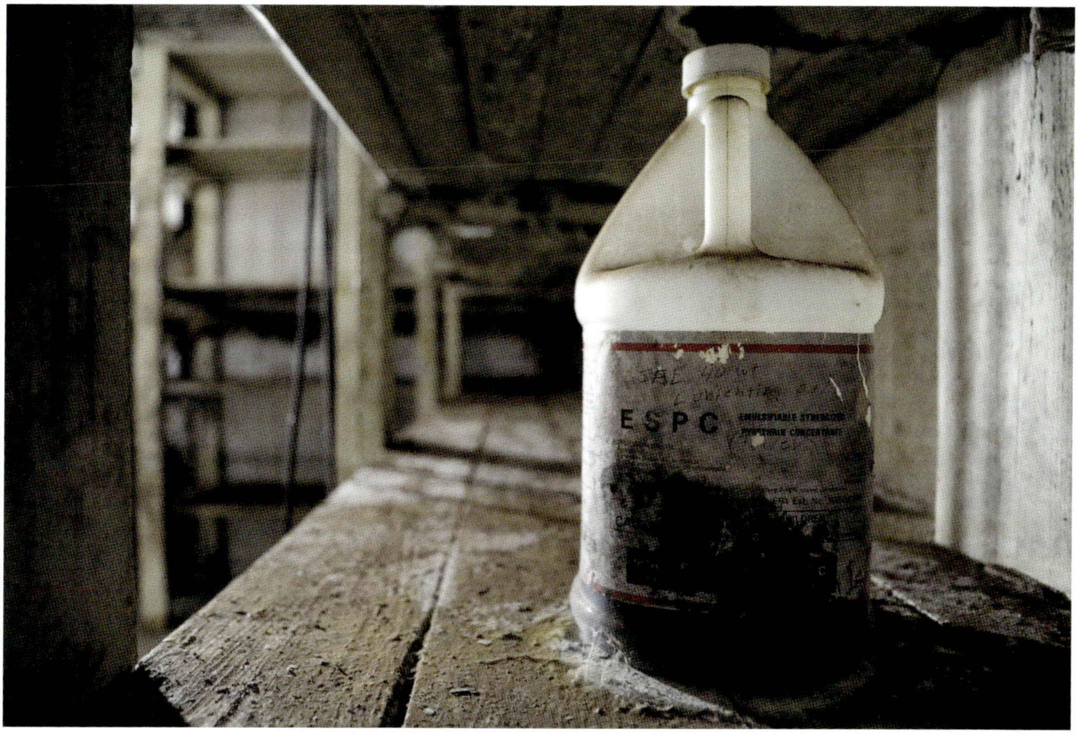

Emulsifiable Synergized Pyrethrin Concentrate (pesticide).

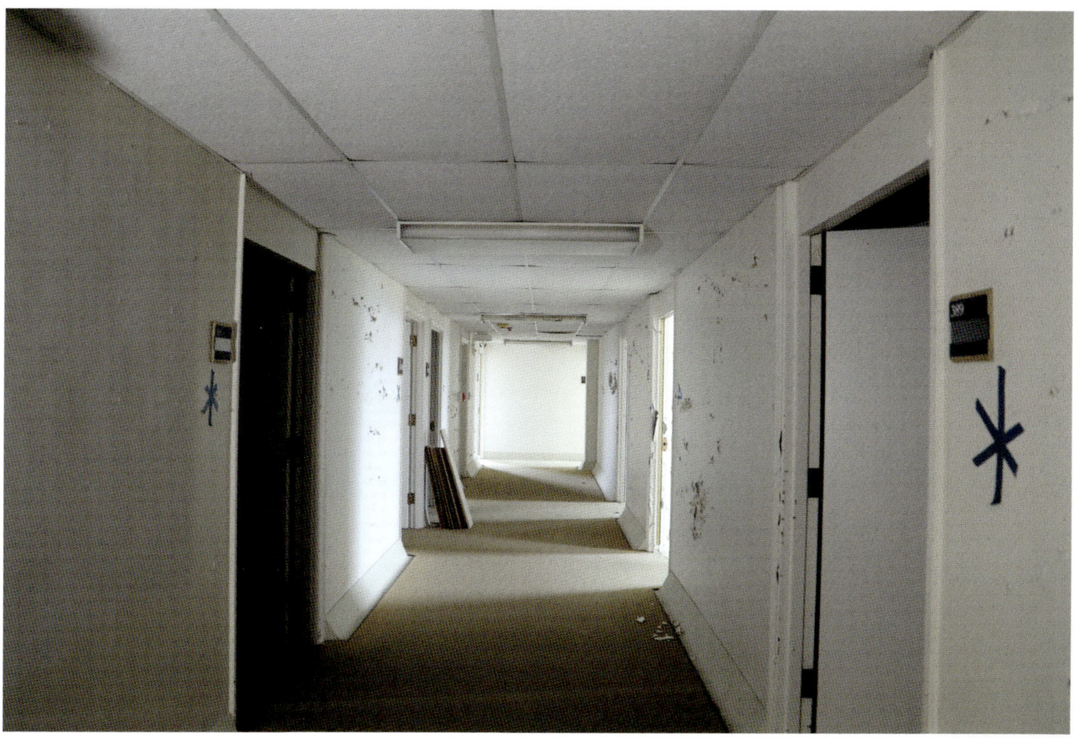

The third floor is in impeccable condition.

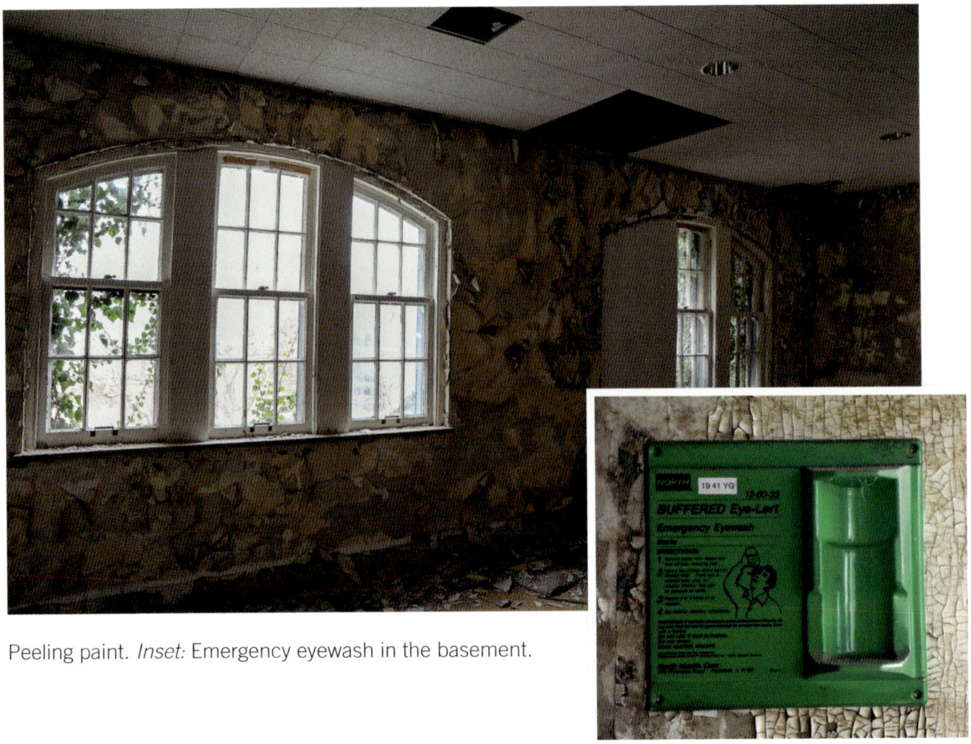

Peeling paint. *Inset:* Emergency eyewash in the basement.

Sunflower Foundation

After a majority of the buildings came down, all that remains on the property is the Main Building with its magnificent clocktower and the old 1921 Power Plant and the 1927 Nurses Dormitory directly across from it. On January 20, 2016, the Sunflower Foundation announced that they had purchased the abandoned nurses' dormitory and powerplant located just down the hill from the clocktower. "For more than a century, Martin's Hill has been a center of pioneering work in health care," said Board Chair Reggie Robinson. "We're thrilled to continue that heritage by establishing a permanent home for the Sunflower Foundation from which it can fulfill its mission to serve as a catalyst for improving the health of all Kansans." The plans for these two buildings are to become the headquarters of the Sunflower Foundation and lease office spaces and conferences for nonprofit organizations. Sunflower's mission is to give grants to further health care incentives in the Sunflower State. This was the start to a very lengthy $12-million project to renovate the buildings that had been abandoned for fifteen years. Having trademarked the term "Healing Hill" for the progressiveness that Menninger's had on mental health and the hopefulness that the Sunflower Foundation will have on healthcare in the future for Topeka residents. Renovations are wrapping up as of summer 2021 and nearing the long-awaited completion of the project.

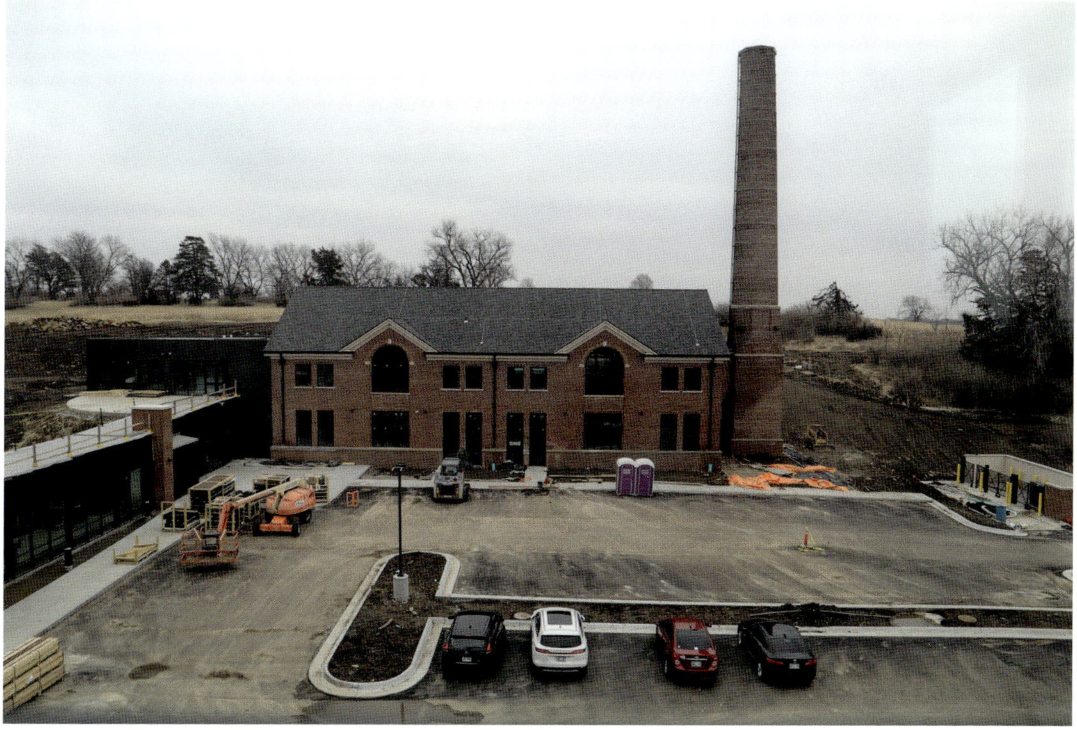

Nurses dormitory and power plant under renovation.

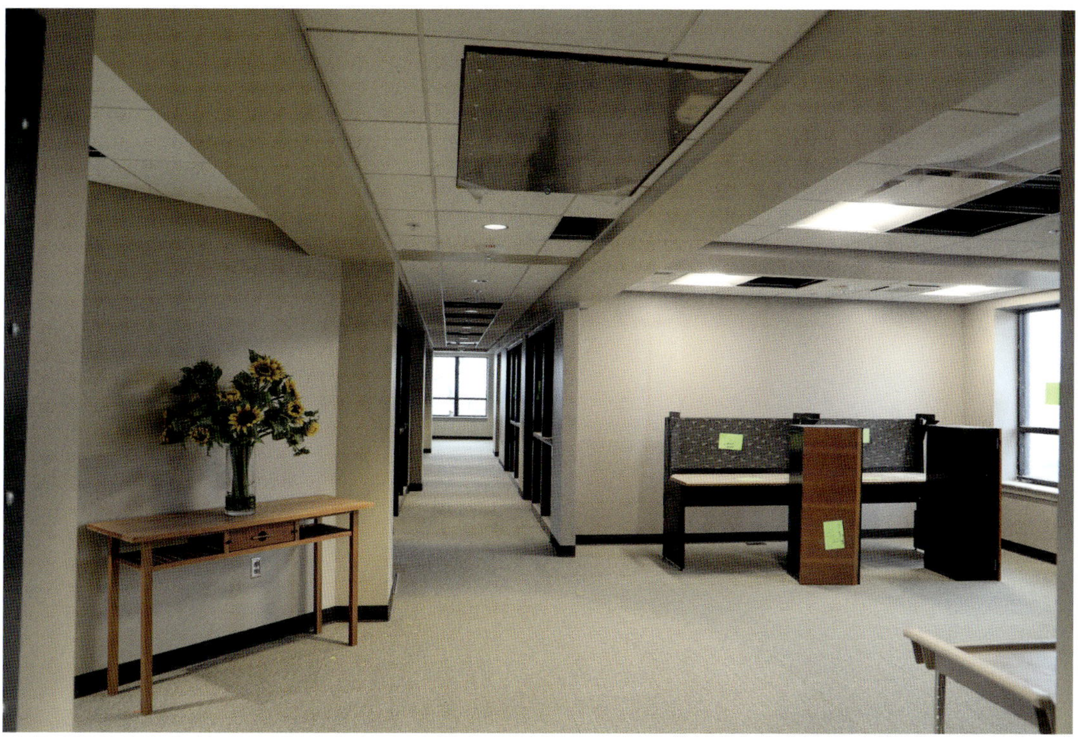

Nurses dormitory top floor.

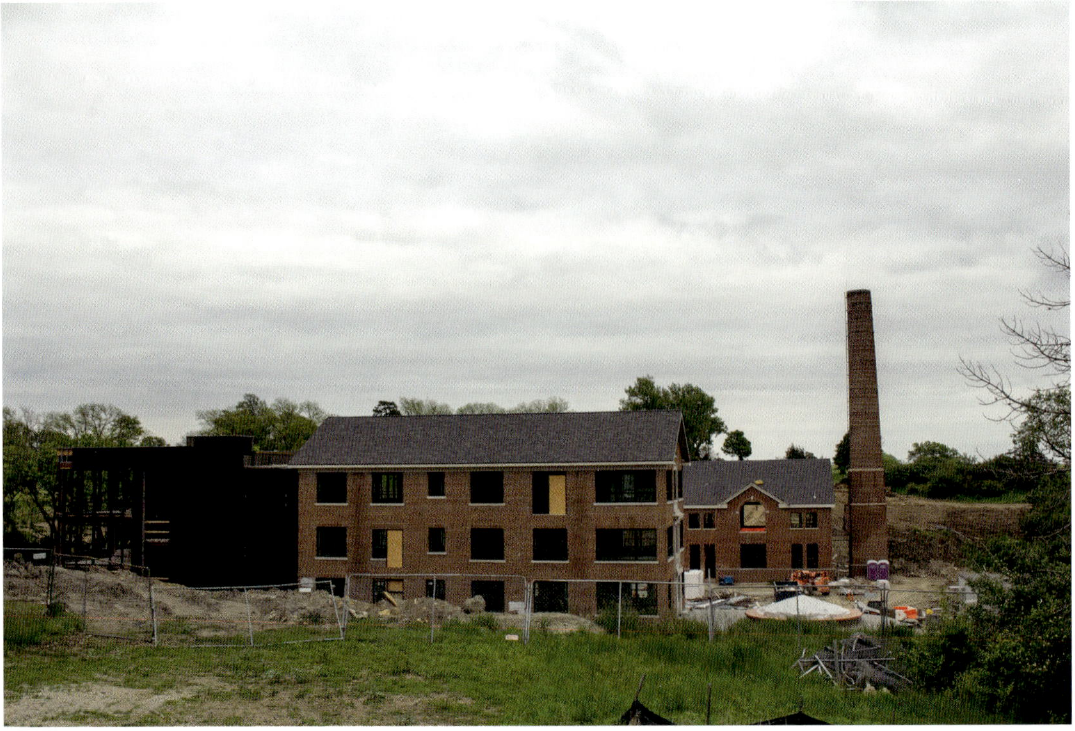

Nurses dormitory and power plant under renovation.

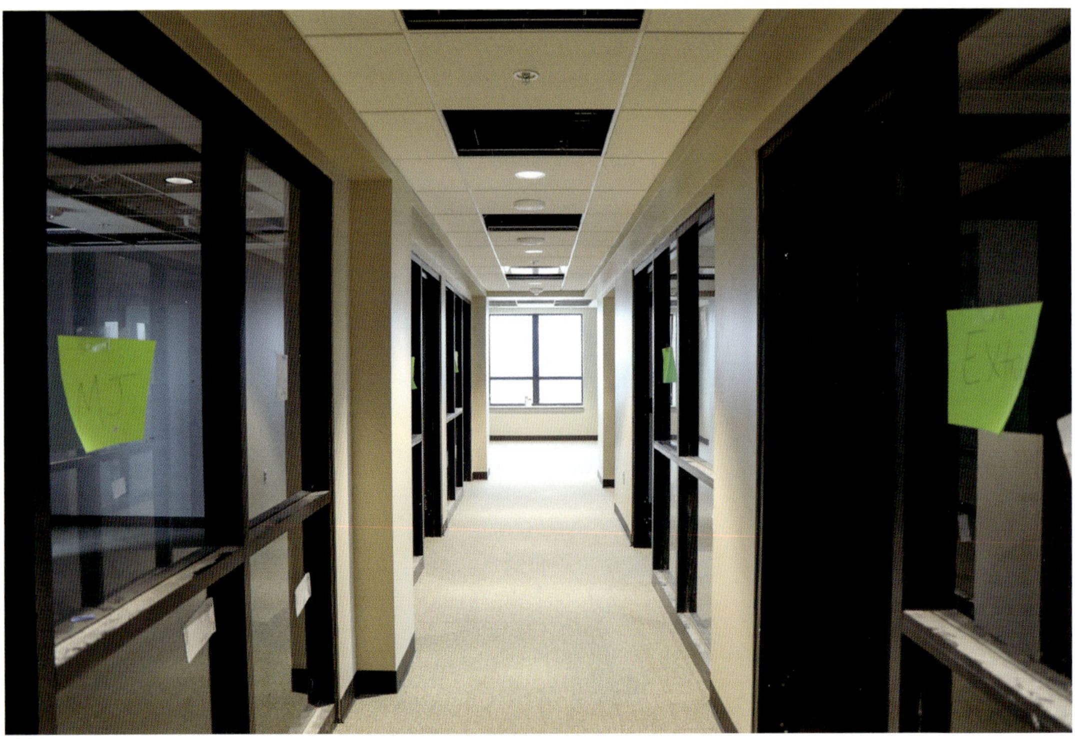

Nurses dormitory top floor.

2

CAPITAL CENTER INN

Holiday Inn City Centre

In 1969, an eight-story, 207-room hotel called the Holiday Inn City Centre was built in the heart of downtown Topeka. The hotel was equipped with a banquet hall, restaurant, cocktail bar, business center, and suites. Amenities included free continental breakfast, plenty of on-site parking, and great guest service. They also offered on-site guest laundry facilities, a game room, an outdoor swimming pool, cable TV with HBO and Showtime, and a lounge for you to relax. The business center could accommodate up to 300 people for conventions or events. All of these perks plus the location generated great clientele.

In 1987, the Holiday Inn made newspaper headlines when a maid went to clean a room around 1:20 p.m. and found the lifeless body of sixty-eight-year-old John R. Stacy. An autopsy reported that the cause of death was suffocation, and his death was being investigated as a homicide. A couple that was seen with Stacy at the hotel were tracked to Missouri and officials said robbery was a possible motive.

Capital Center Inn/Red Carpet Inn & Suites

In the late 1990s/early 200s, the hotel went by Capital Center Inn and Red Carpet Inn & Suites, both used interchangeably. It hosted many lavish conferences, events, and served those visiting the Golden City. But a few short years later on June 17, 2005, the cocktail lounge on the eighth floor fell victim to an arson fire. All patrons were evacuated safely, but it ultimately led to the closure of the hotel. It sat abandoned for many years and continued to suffer at the hands of vandalism and break-ins, causing the entire building to be gutted.

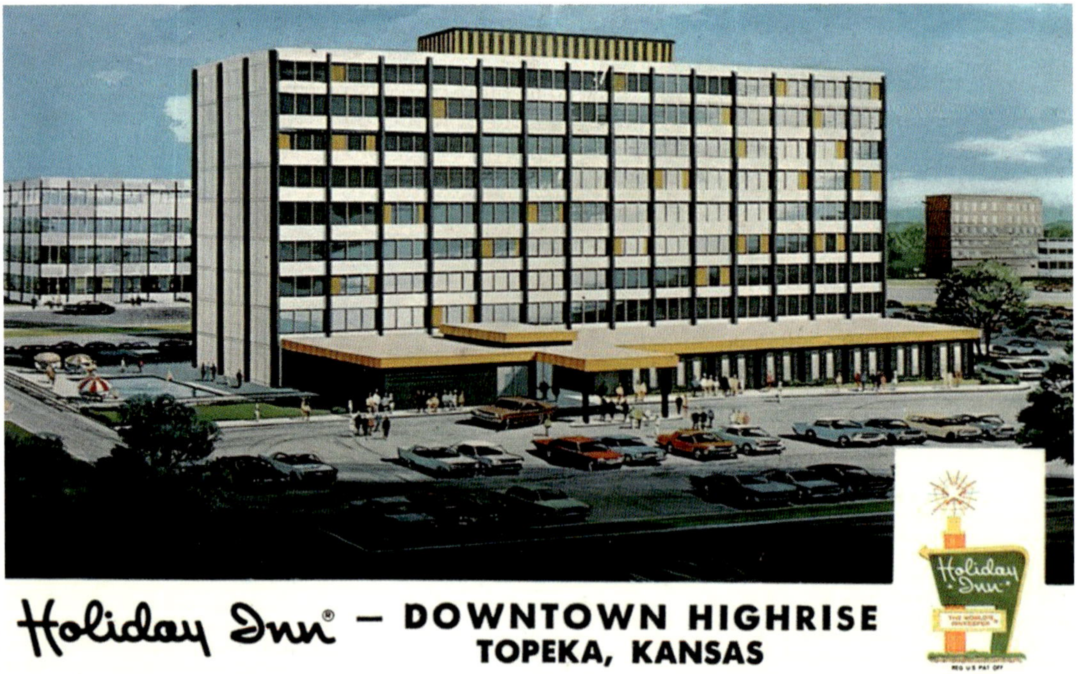

Holiday Inn postcard *ca*. 1970s.

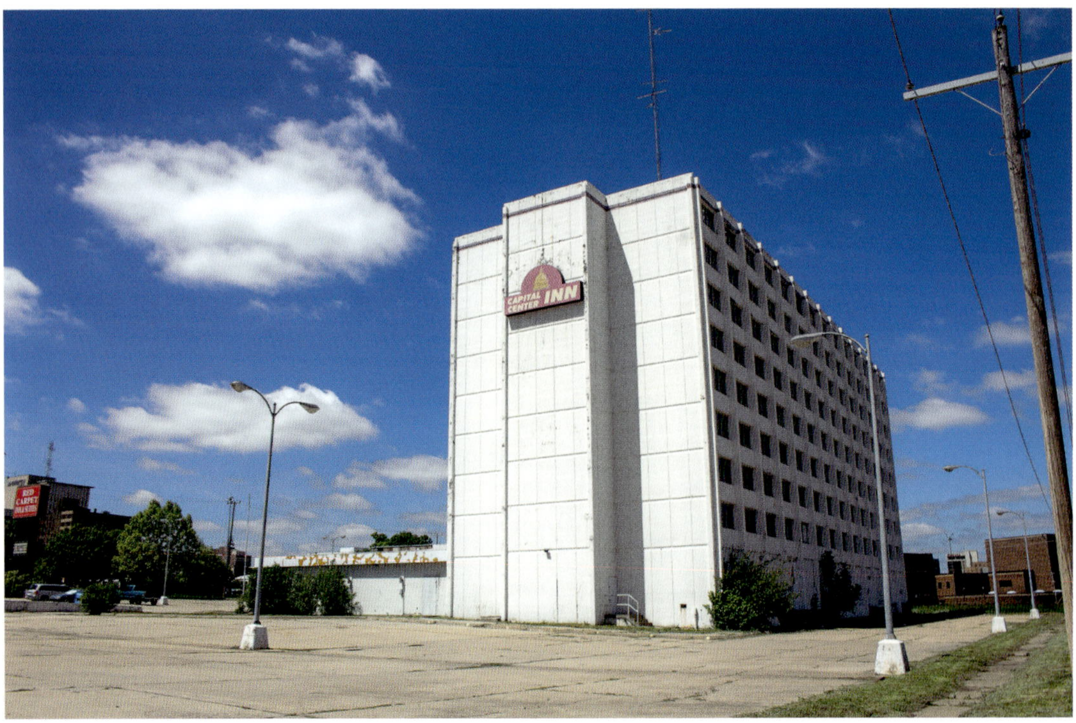

View from the street.

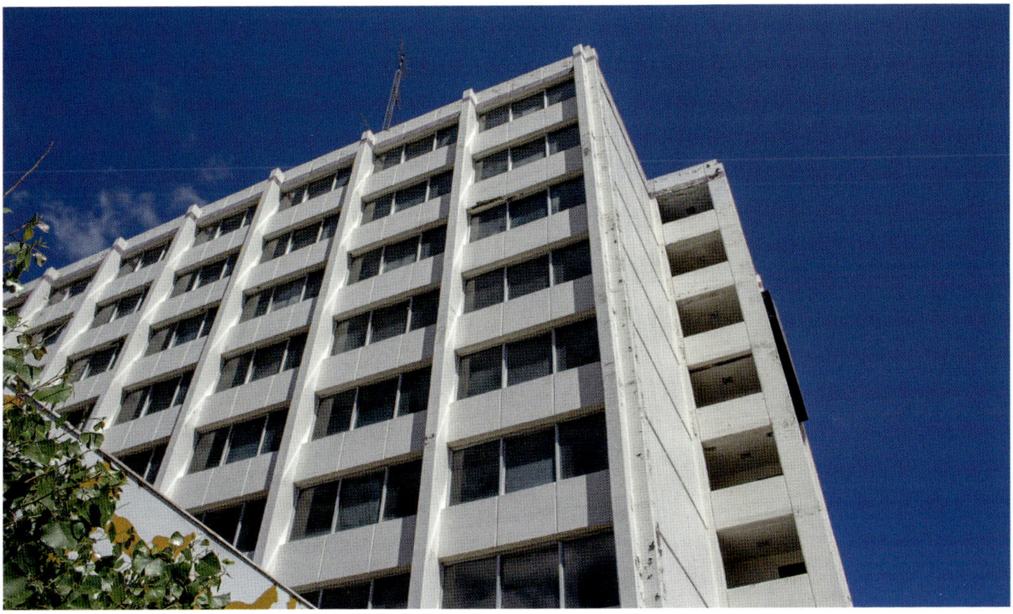

Most windows on all eight-stories are still intact.

An eight-man crew with Mcpherson Wrecking Inc. started work in February 2011 to gut the hotel due to the ongoing break-ins and vandalism. On average it took about two weeks to gut one floor, putting the project at a timeline of around sixteen-to-eighteen weeks to complete. Mcpherson usually sells scrap metal they remove from structures, but the Capital Center Inn had already had most of its copper stripped by thieves, even stripping the elevator shaft. Further evidence showed homeless activity, but despite being abandoned for six years at the time, Mcpherson said the structure appeared to be in pretty fair condition. It is unclear if this assessment is still to be true now that it has been abandoned for fifteen years and is starting to lose stucco from the top floors.

In recent years, the City of Topeka has entered into a battle for backed taxes on the building. The owner had typically been respectful about catching up on payments and bringing things up to code when brought to his attention. But he has since fallen behind on three years' worth of property taxes, fines, and maintenance done on the property, totaling a bill of $102,059. Over the last eight years, the property has accumulated over forty violations, including landscaping, graffiti, and safety violations.

"To mow the property ranges from $250 to $350 and the same for sanitation depending on the amount of debris that we had to pick up and after the first violation of the year and an administrative penalty that starts out at $100 which is just part of the fine increased to $200 if we have to do it more than once," said one person. The property as of 2020 is valued at around $690,000 decreasing with each passing year, the future of it is uncertain.

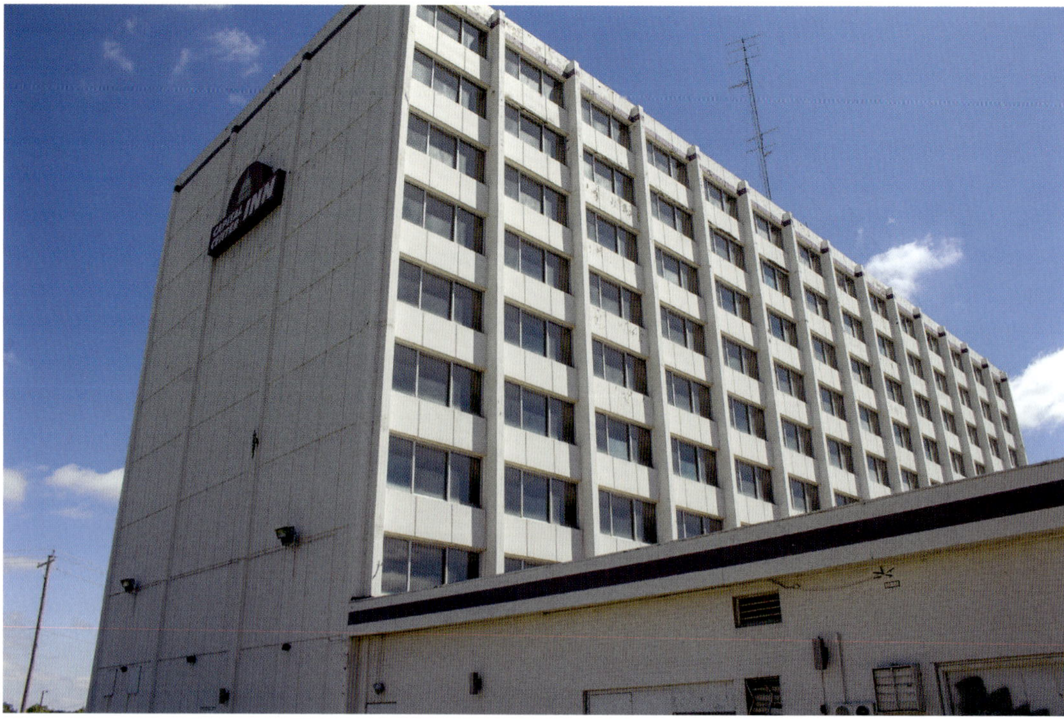

This side of the once luxury hotel now faces the Shawnee County Correctional Facility.

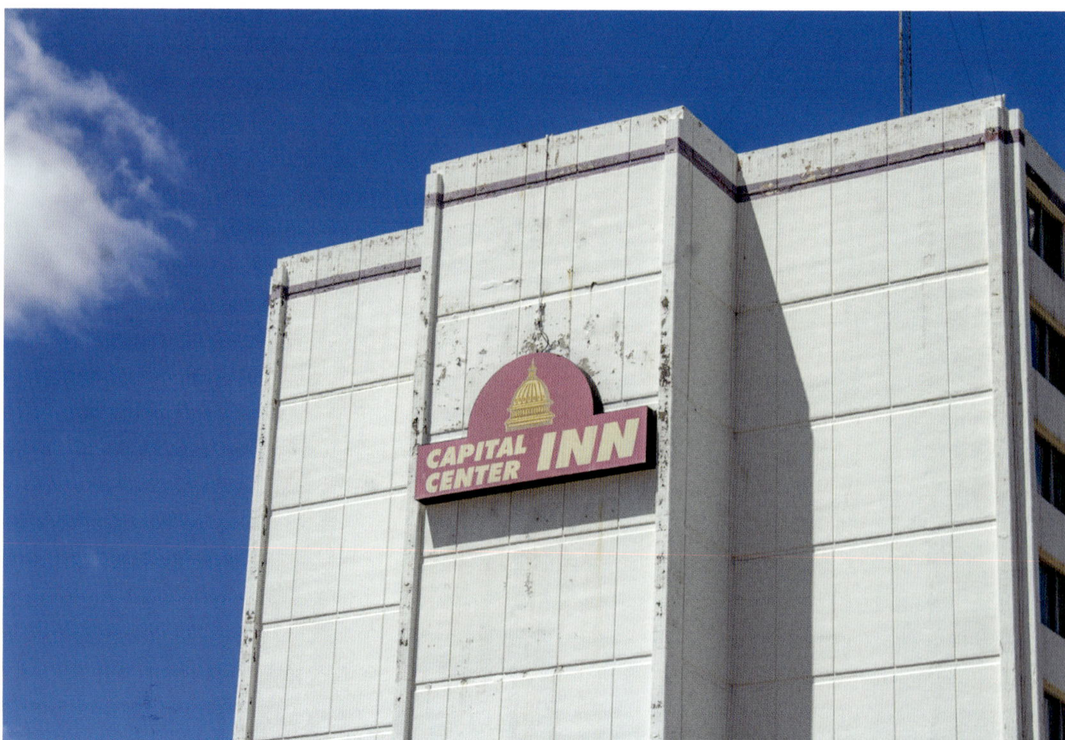

Capital Center Inn.

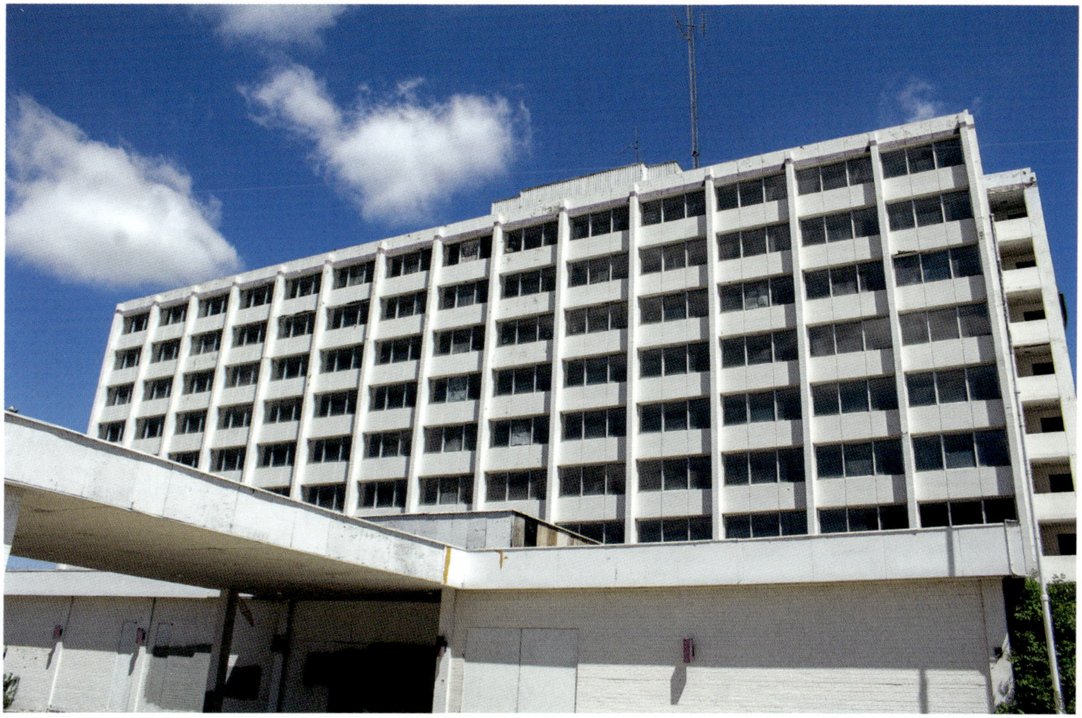

Drive-through entryway.

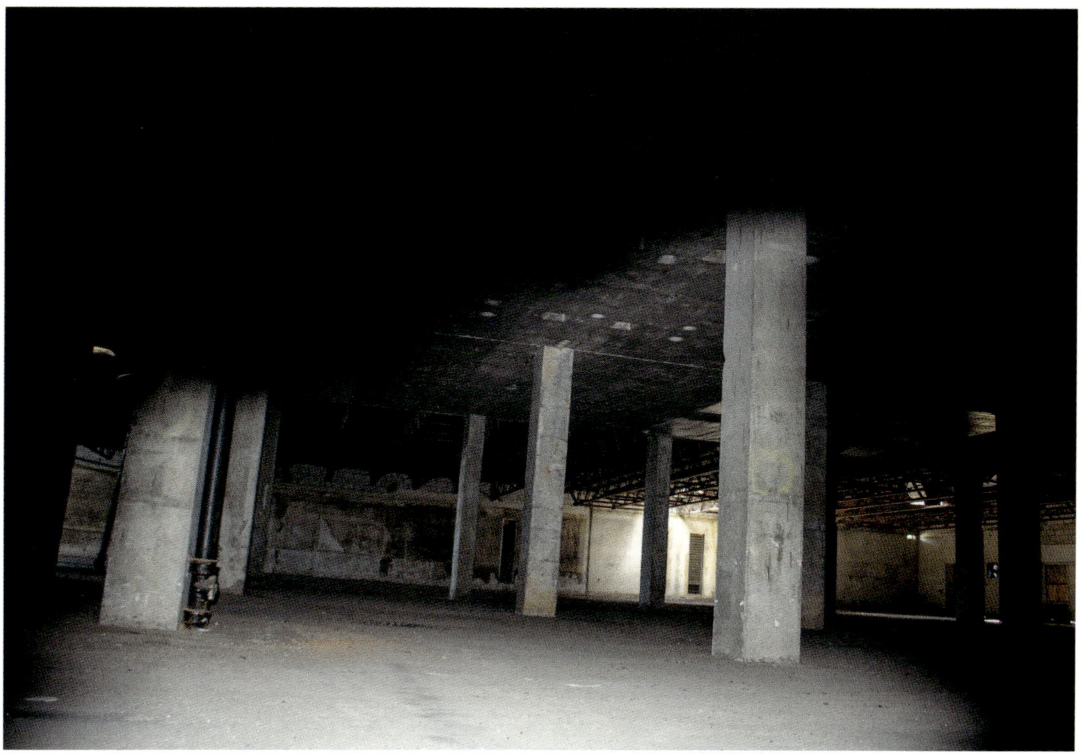

Interior completely gutted and stripped.

3

McKINLEY ELEMENTARY SCHOOL

McKinley Elementary School was one of the four all-Black elementary schools in Topeka. The other three were Buchanan, Washington, and Monroe, which has now been turned into the Brown v. Board of Education National Historic Site.

Lane School

The history of the McKinley school and property dates back to 1879, before it was McKinley at all. It got its start as a small district one-room schoolhouse with about thirty-to-forty students attending and one teacher. In order to progress with growing attendance, three wings were added to create four classrooms in 1882 and the name "Lane School" was picked out for the building. Professor S. G. Watkins was given the role as the first principal of the growing student body. Students would attend K-6th grade and would then transfer to the nearby Grant or Quincy schools for their continued education.

McKinley Grade School

Around 1905, a petition from students, parents, and teachers started circulating to build a grander and more accommodating school, thus becoming McKinley Grade School. Lundgren & Carlson Contractors were hired for the project and construction was underway from 1906-07. It finished at a final cost of $24,922, allowing for students to begin classes in the new building in 1908. The new building had six classrooms, two floors, and boasted around 175 students, five teachers, a principal, and a janitor. Kindergarten through eighth grade in North Topeka would attend here and after graduation often attended Quincy Junior High.

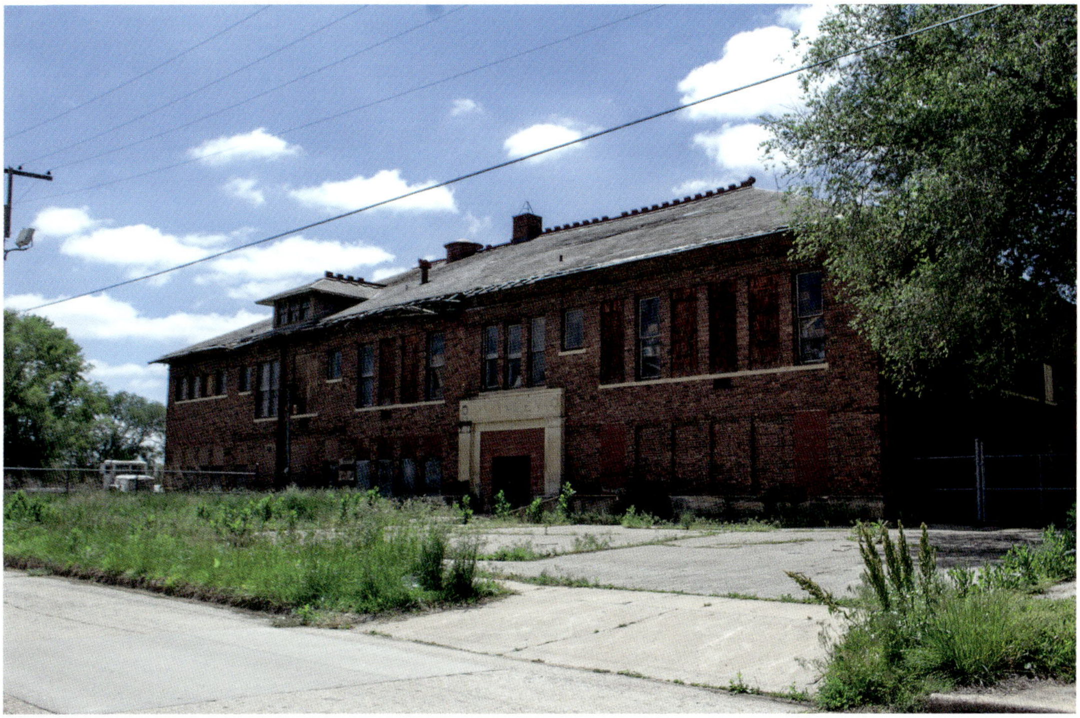

Street view of McKinley Grade School.

Just a few years later it was evident that the overcrowding in the third ward school was out of hand with 306 students. McKinley was the source of the most severe overcrowding in the district, not allowing any enrollments past the sixth grade for a short time, and even for lower grades, most had to be transferred to one of the other three remaining African American elementary schools. A resolution was passed giving $11,950 for an addition of four rooms, heating, ventilation, and remodeling the older portion of the building. This was not the end of the problems in regard to the building's condition, with more concerns being raised. It was brought to the attention of the school board in July 1914 that two of the rooms in the school had never been floored, the playground was much too small and that no sewers were present in the facility, making sanitary conditions unacceptable. The school board knew this was an issue that needed to be fixed as soon as possible, but the city water department made things less than easy. They refused to extend water main lines two blocks to reach McKinley unless the board ensured they received $63 a year for two years. After years of negotiations and meetings, Wilbur Stanfield agreed to extend the lines to the school, giving the students water fountains and indoor restrooms.

McKinley was one of the best schools within the entire Topeka district providing outstanding education for its students. It also providing many events and sports for the kids to get involved in including baseball, basketball, girl reserves, etc. The school continued to grow, receiving numerous additions to try and cope with the influx of students always coming in as the third ward community grew. Another one of those additions came in 1926 with the contract being let to J. A. Black for $21,701.12.

Harrison Caldwell became the superintendent of Topeka's four all-Black elementary schools in 1941. He was known as a hard worker, very involved in the community and schools, and excelled at his job. At the time he took over, he oversaw almost thirty teachers and around 900 students. Linda and Terry Brown of the famous Brown v. Board of Education case and the Sumner School attended McKinley Elementary School for a while when their father was assigned to the nearby St. Mark AME Church. The school was highly reputable in their education, morals, and the students they put into the world.

Former student Carolyn Campbell said with pride:

> I am thankful to share my journey that began as a proud product of segregation. Of all four Black elementary schools (Monroe, Buchanan, Washington, and McKinley), my home away from home was McKinley Elementary in North Topeka. At McKinley, we were educated, nurtured, and valued. Every day we stepped through the doors, well-educated, strict but caring Black teachers stressed excellence. I hope I am making it clear there were high expectations, our teachers saw potential in each of us. Ethel Williams Barbour was our principal, she had a beautiful smile and nurturing spirit. Mr. McDonald was our kind custodian, and my next-door neighbor, Geraldine Harmon, was my second-grade teacher. My mama had to tell me that I couldn't call her Jerry at school. One of the life skills we were taught was saving money. There was an actual bank modeled after real banks, and we could open a savings account.

Palmer Blackwell gave his account of relying on teachers for more than education, "The teacher Mrs. Monroe would come to my house and pick me up and take me to school," he remembered.

During the tragic flood of 1951, North Topeka had gotten hit pretty badly, causing many students to be transferred to the Buchanan Elementary School. It wasn't but a few years later that the landmark decision of the Supreme Court in the Brown v. Board of Education caused many schools to close, desegregate, and consolidate in Topeka. McKinley was one of the schools to close shortly after at the end of 1954 due to Topeka's new neighborhood school district plans, unlike the Monroe & Buchanan Elementary School, schools that were able to be restored into functional facilities once again.

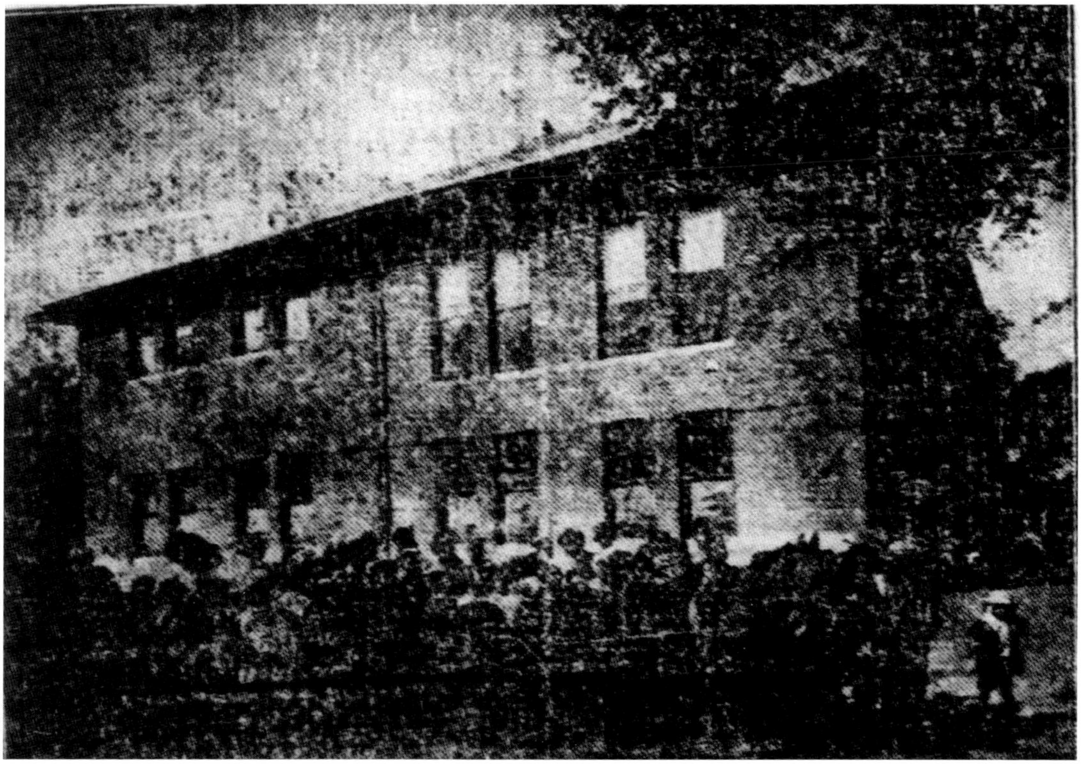

African American McKinley School. [*The Topeka Daily Capital, October 7, 1908*]

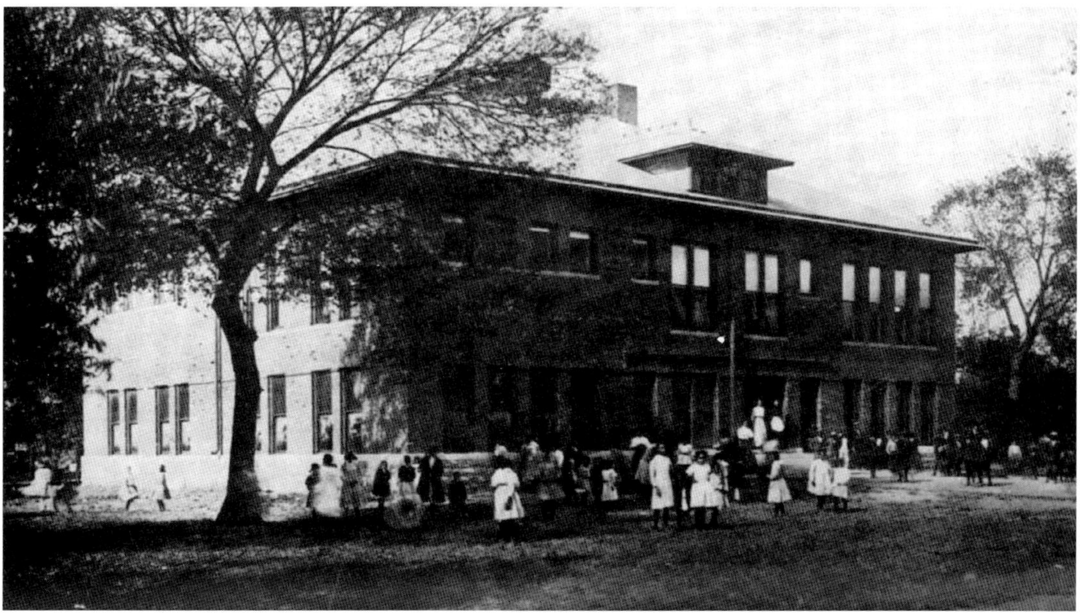

McKinley Elementary School *ca.* 1911. [*Topeka Public Schools Annual Report*]

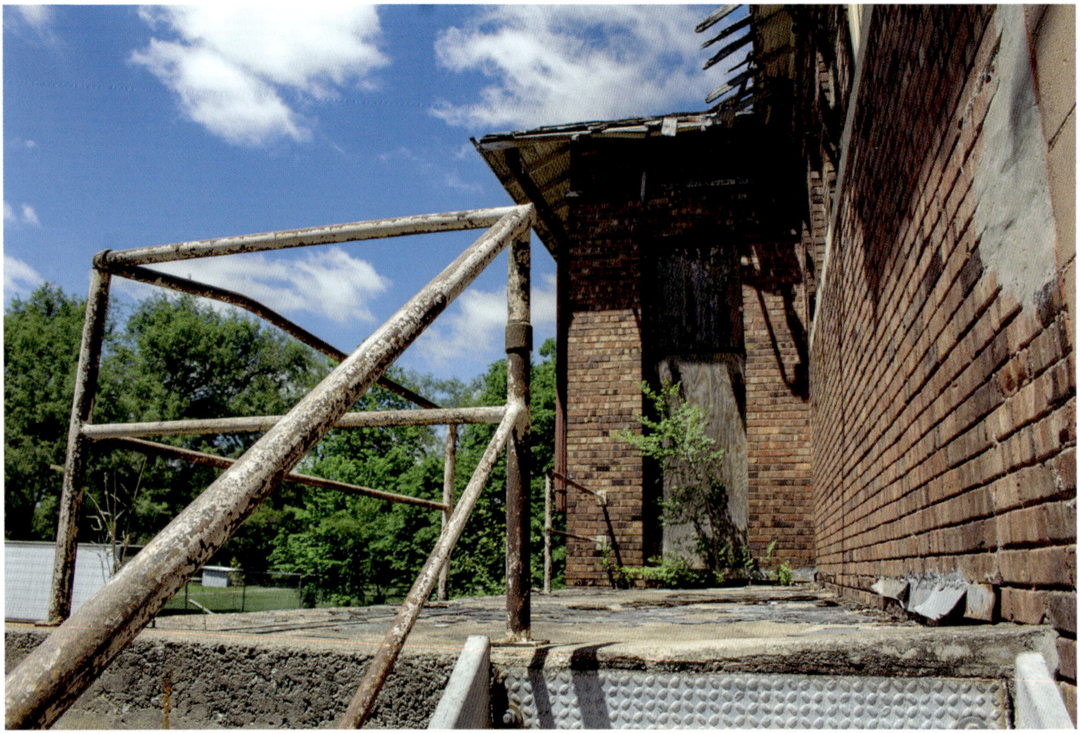

Stairway on the backside of the school.

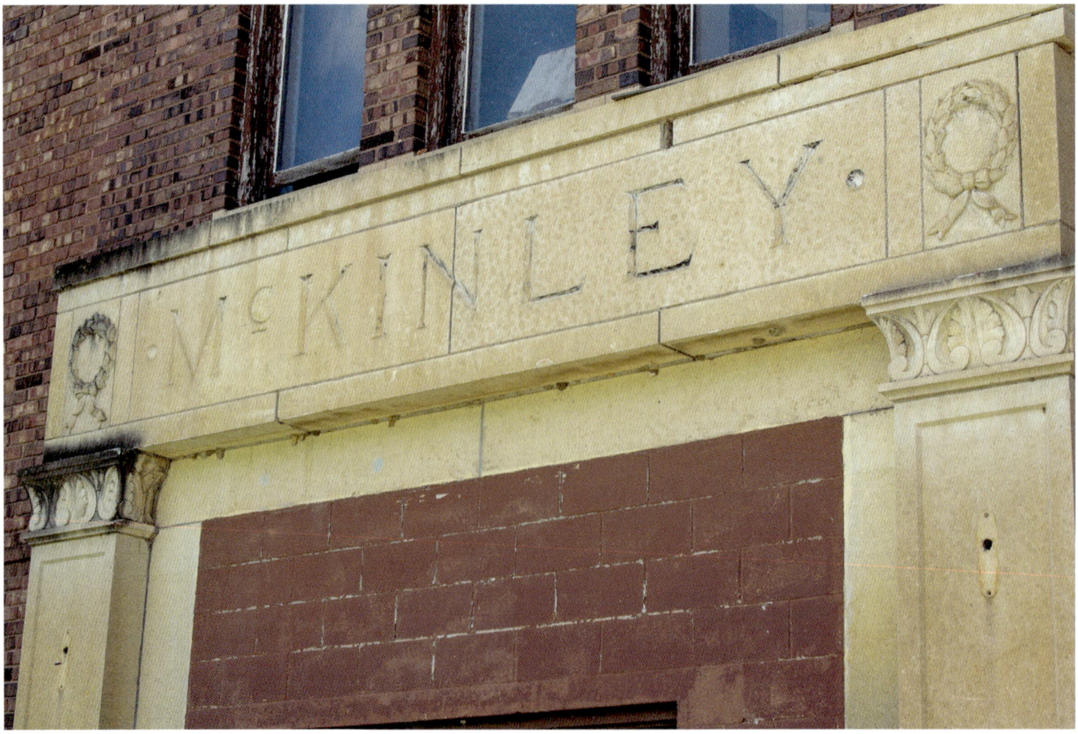

Entrance to McKinley Elementary School.

Right: Upper-kindergarten girls ready for a fairy dance. Lower: Editorial staff of the *McKinley Breeze.* [*The Topeka Daily Capital, November 16, 1919*]

Below: Every room is now used as storage, filled almost to the top with things.

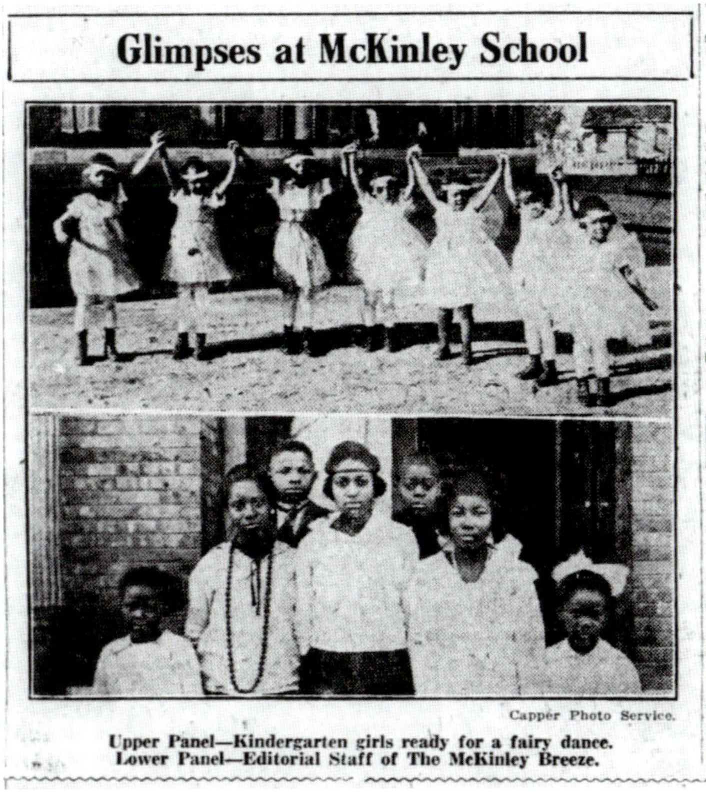

Glimpses at McKinley School

Capper Photo Service.

Upper Panel—Kindergarten girls ready for a fairy dance.
Lower Panel—Editorial Staff of The McKinley Breeze.

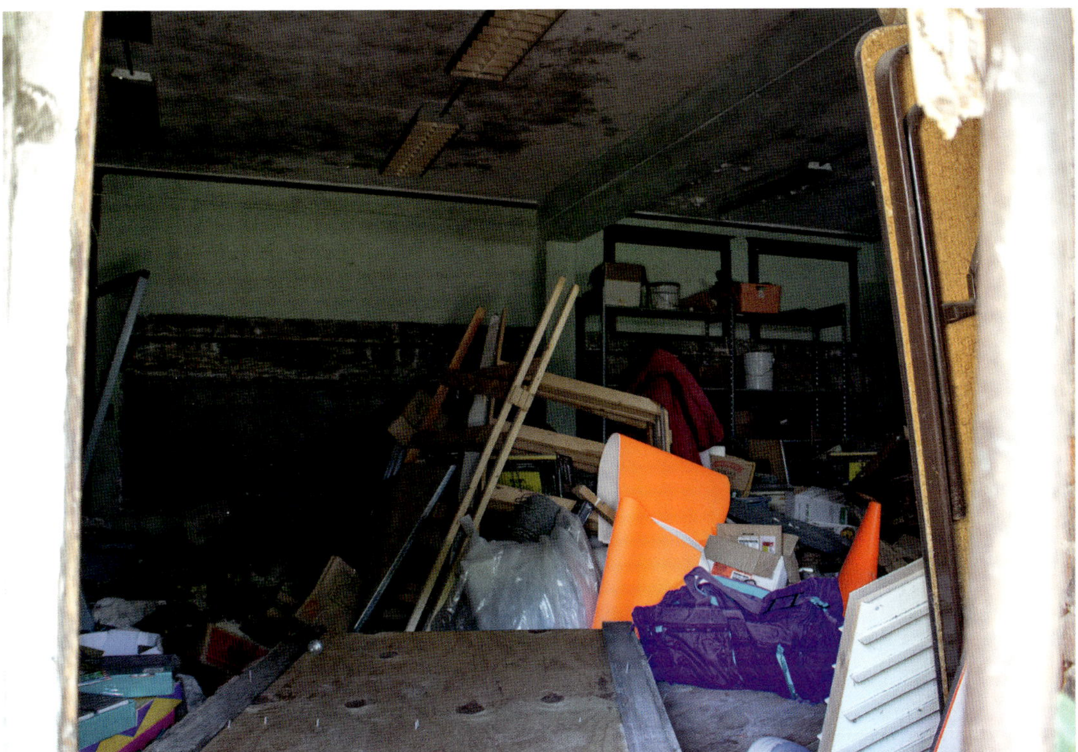

Monroe Elementary became the Brown v. Board of Education National Historic Site ran by the National Park Service. Buchanan Elementary was renovated to become the Housing and Credit Counseling, Inc. facility. McKinley and Sumner, the school at the center of the Brown v. Board of Education case, sit and further deteriorate. The McKinley school is and has been used as storage for many years, but according to the owner has suffered at the hands of multiple break-ins where vandals have stolen and damaged many items inside.

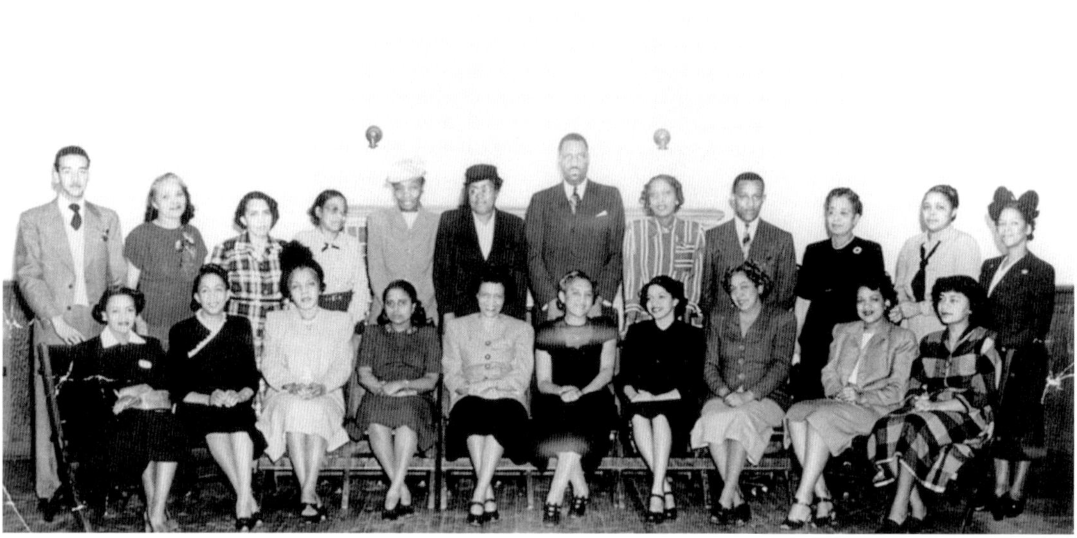

Teachers of the four all-Black schools in 1949. Standing left to right: Merrill Ross, Myrtle Starnes, Edna Vance, Fannie Palton, Mamie Williams, Eva Walker, Harrison Caldwell (superintendent), Ehtel Barbour (principal of McKinley), J. B. Holland, Ida Norman (school nurse), Althea McBrier. Seated from left to right: Katherine King, Dorothy Bradshaw, Mildred North, Geraldine Gilliam, Minerva Washington, Ada Eggleston, Barbara Ross, Dorothy Crawford, Doris Love, Julia Patterson. [*Courtesy of Dr. Owen M. Henson*]

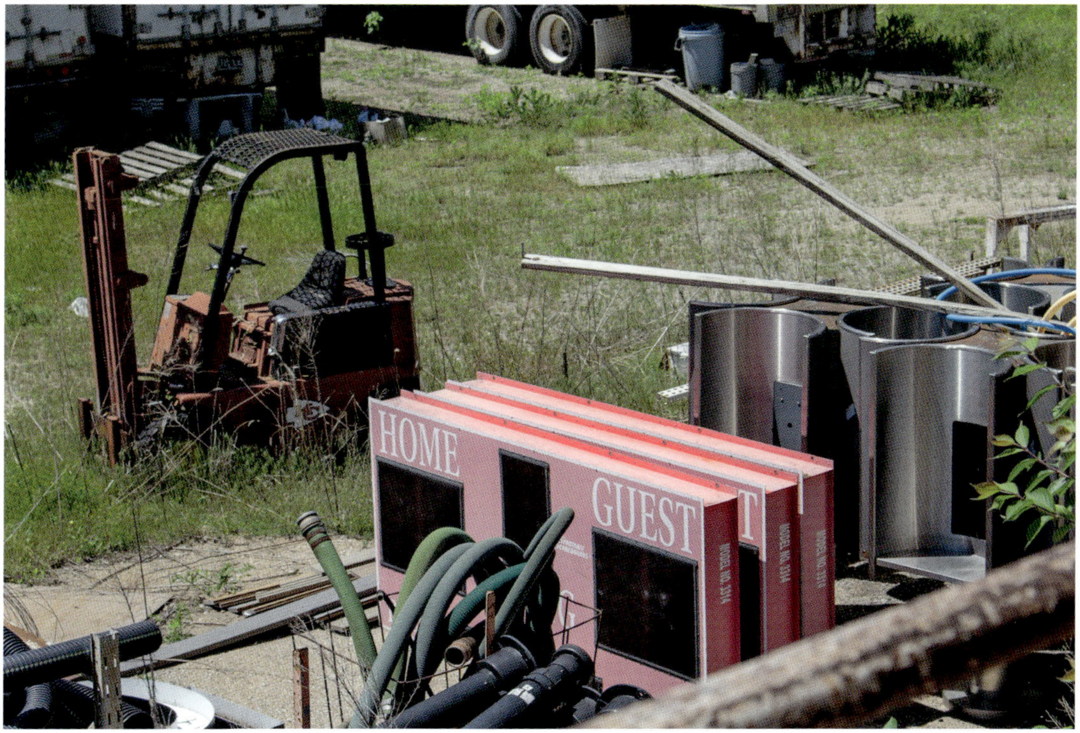

The rest of the playground now displays a collection of items such as these scoreboards.

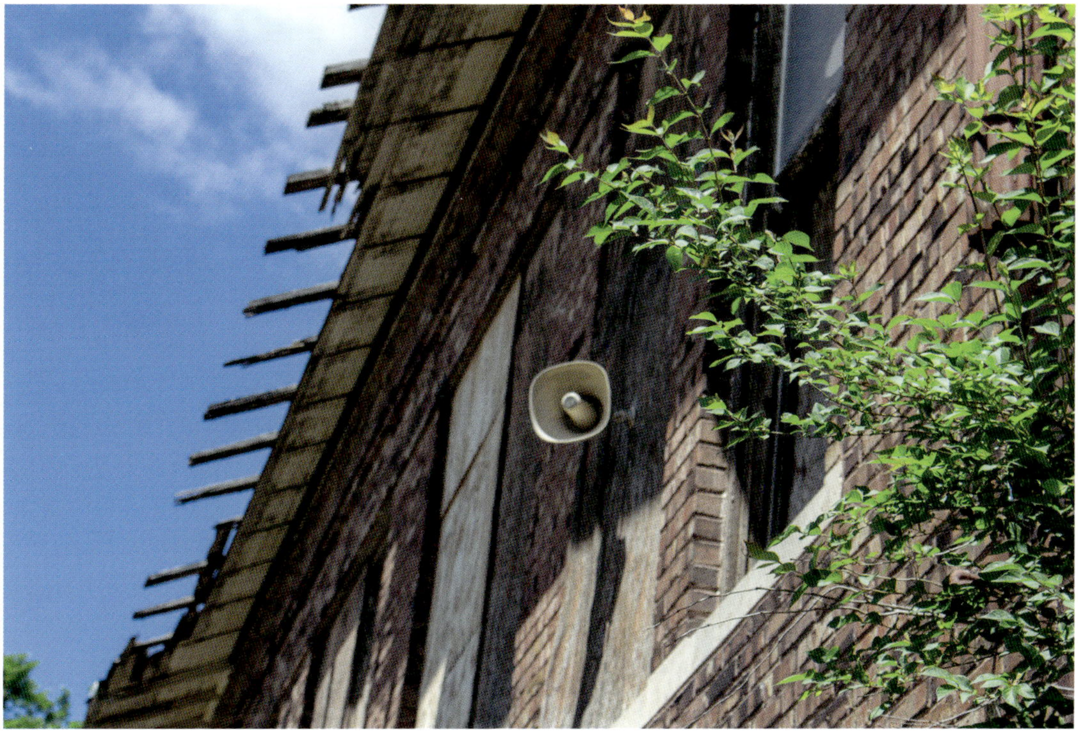

Was this speaker used to call students in from recess?

4

SUMNER ELEMENTARY SCHOOL

1880-1894 First Sumner School

The first Sumner School was built in the fourth ward as a two-story, four-room brick schoolhouse. It was completed at a cost of $6,000 with a belfry in the center and was ready for occupancy in October 1880. At the time it was the school the African American children in the district attended and was involved in a court case a few months after opening. For the same reasons it would later make national headlines. The case of *Eveline Phillips v. The Board of Education of Topeka* was filed in district court in November 1880. The Plaintiffs, James Phillips on behalf of his two children, hired Rossington & Smith and H. P. Dillion, attorneys, and D. A. Harvey, attorney, for the defense, the Board of Education of Topeka. The Plaintiffs argued that they were refused instruction by the teacher of the Clay Street School per order of the Board of Education of Topeka who directed that they attend the Sumner School, which was set apart for African American students. James Phillips said the Sumner School was a considerable distance from their house.

What started off as a school to educate Black children was turned into an all-White school in 1885. The reasoning was changing boundaries of the school district. First through fifth grade White students would attend Sumner School now with D. C. Tillotson as the superintendent. The Black students were moved out and taught in a smaller two-room frame building close by. This building suffered severe wind damage that blew the roof in during the spring of 1896 and was rebuilt as a one-story frame building. Tragedy struck on November 12, 1894, when a fire broke out in the Sumner School, causing nearly $8,000 worth of damage. Fierce winds blew that evening, causing the fire to spread quickly and be visible from streets over. A crowd of dozens started to gather, watching the very first Sumner School as it burned

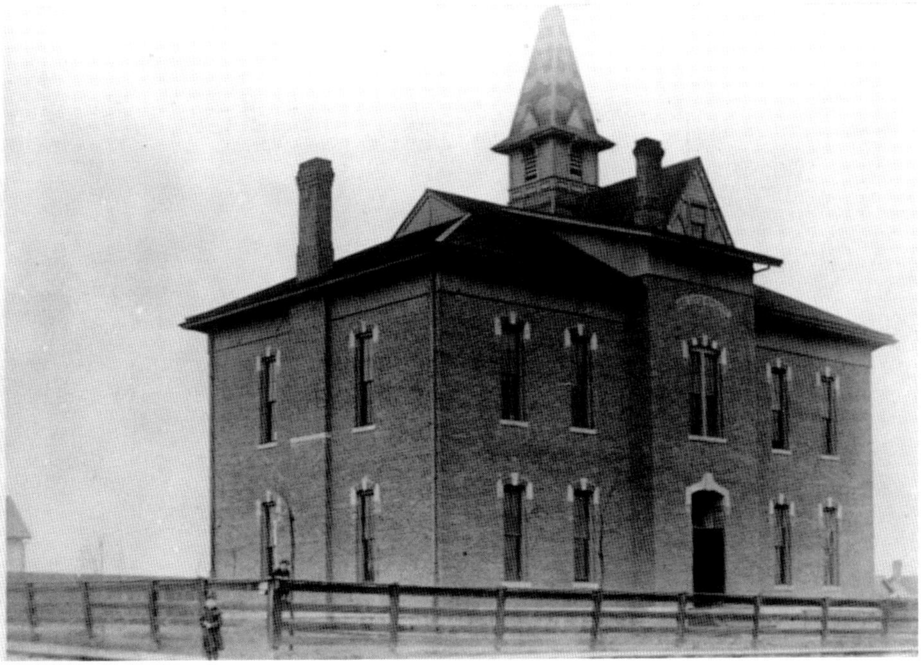

First Sumner School *ca.* 1885-1894. [*Herbert Ragsdale*]

entirely, far too gone to be saved at all. The fire was first discovered by janitor William Page as he was sweeping an upstairs room but managed to make it out safely. The building was only insured for $2,000 and after a thorough investigation, the school board decided to use the gutted building because of its still standing brick walls. Students would attend Douglas School a few streets over until repairs were complete.

1894-1899 "Second" Sumner School

Architect T. H. Lescher gave an estimate for his work amounting to $2,500, just $500 over what insurance would cover. Plans would be made up and bids would be advertised ensuring that work would be completed as soon as possible. James Fitzgibbons was hired to bolt the walls to ensure their safety, with bolts that were forty feet long. A new roof was put on and the four classrooms rebuilt, allowing for classes to commence the following semester. School for the next two years went on as normal until parents of students started noticing a growing crack in the bricks. The whole building started to have a crooked appearance and a wall began to buckle. Parents and children were told not to worry and that a thorough investigation was conducted deeming the building safe as ever. But it was decided to fix the growing crack anyways. Bricks were taken out of place and anchored securely as well as iron bars placed lengthwise of the building.

Just a year later, the school board could no longer outrun the inevitable: Sumner School must be torn down and rebuilt from the ground up. After numerous repairs and efforts to prolong having to build a new school, there were no further repairs that could be done while still keeping the integrity of a safe building. J. S. Morse was the leading bid with $267 to tear down the old building. Students were transferred to Jackson and Douglas Schools for the next two years while the new building was being constructed.

1901-1936 Third Sumner School

The third Sumner School was agreed to be built in 1900 and the following year bids were taken on the building and its amenities. After $40,000, the brand-new two-story brick building with twelve classrooms was completed in the spring of 1902. Capacity of the modern educational facility would accommodate about 600-700 students and went from first to eighth grade. Architect H. M. Hadley drew up the plans and Cuthbert & Sargent were hired as the contractors. The main entrance on the west side of the building led to a large main hallway, a main stairway divided on a landing into two with one stairway going left and the other going right. Floors and stairs were made of the best hard maple with white enameled wainscoting along the hallways and stairways. The second floor included a large assembly room with seating for 100 pupils.

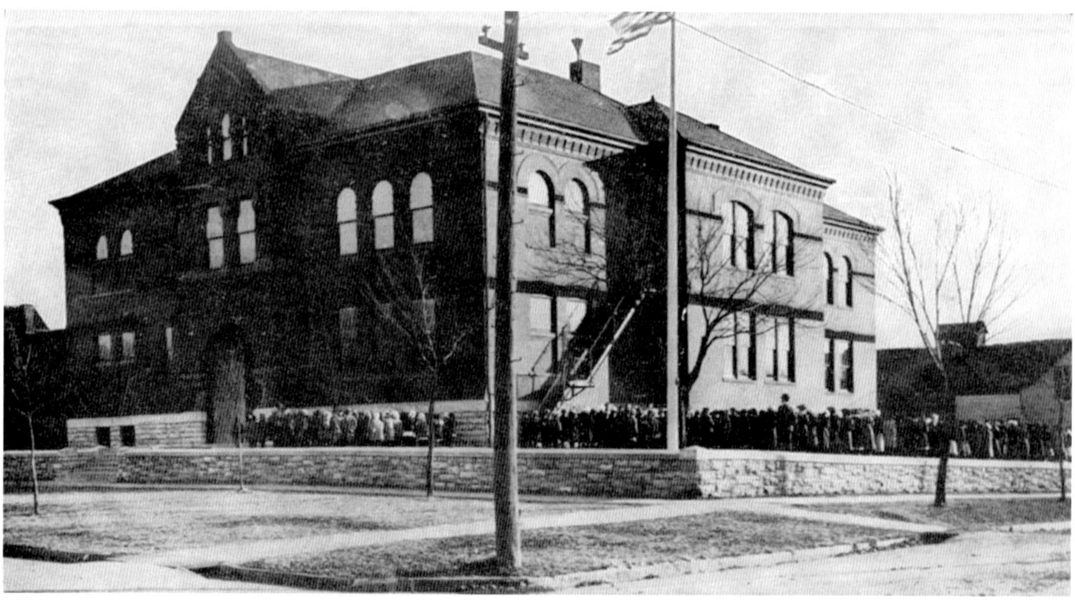

Third Sumner School. [*John F. Strickrott, 1902*]

Third Sumner School was the first school in Topeka to experiment with a music program dedicating a room entirely to music in 1906. In addition, other programs included woodcarving, track, baseball, basketball, and eventually a paper and a very popular flower club. In the 1920s, a ninth grade was added to Sumner, incorporating a full junior high in addition to it being an elementary school. This third building was in use until around 1935, when a new fourth Sumner School was being constructed. There was no need for the old building anymore and it was demolished. A plaque was put on the new building commemorating the replacement of the 1901 school.

1936-1996 Fourth Sumner School

All four Sumner Schools have been on the same lot since 1880 when the first building was built. Sumner Elementary School was built in 1935-36 at around $50,000 as a two-story brick elementary school that served kindergarten through sixth grade. Thomas W. Williamson designed it as an elegant, art deco, renaissance-styled school and with the help of the Federal Emergency Administration of Public Works New Deal program. The layout originally had thirteen rooms, but after undergoing multiple renovations over the years now has seventeen rooms. These include ten classrooms, industrial arts rooms, a clinic, teachers' lounge, administrative offices, and a multi-purpose auditorium. The auditorium had a basement beneath it where during the wintertime P.E. classes would be held. The cafeteria was located in the basement as well. At the time it was built it was still only serving White students of the fourth ward. African American elementary students went to one of four schools Monroe, Buchanan, McKinley, and Washington.

In 1951, Linda Brown, a third grader at Monroe, and her parents, attempted to enroll her at the closer Sumner Elementary School, but her application was denied due to racial segregation. This led to the historic case of *Brown v. Board of Education.*

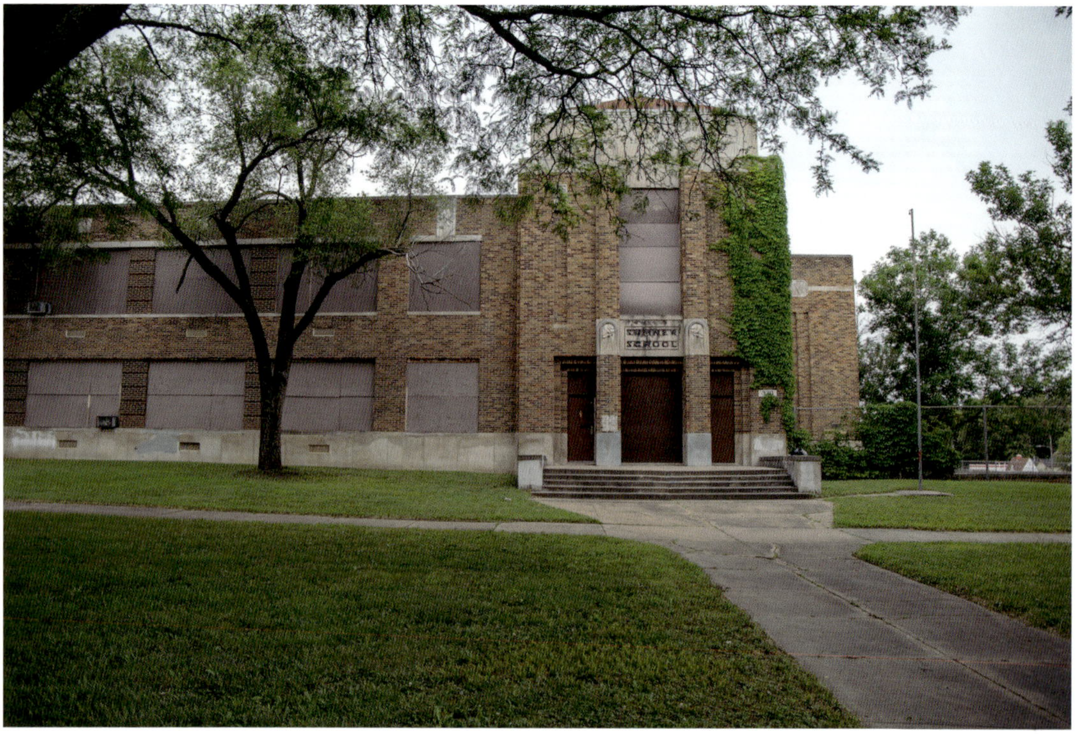

Fourth Sumner Elementary School.

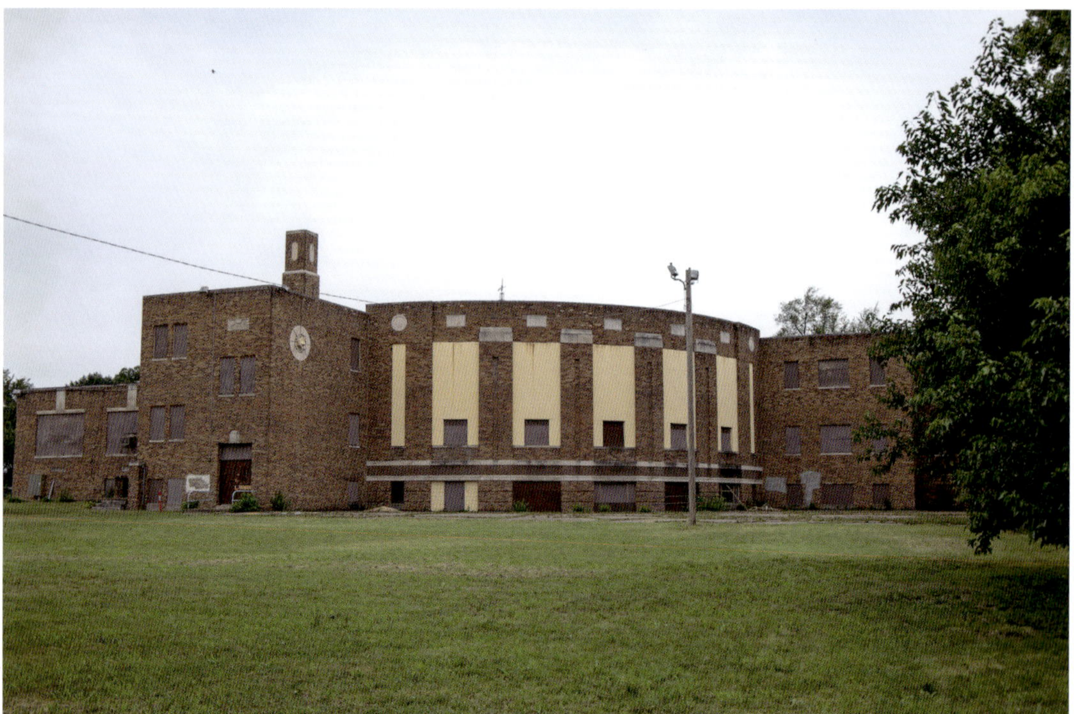

Backside of Sumner Elementary showing rounded auditorium.

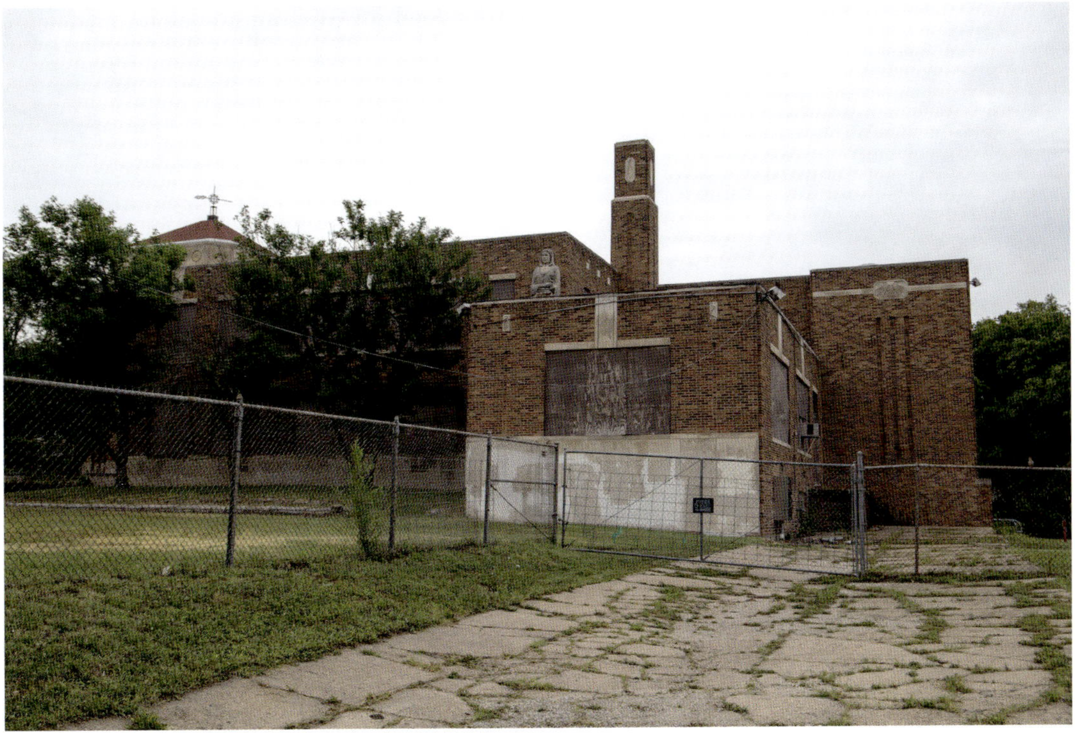

Mother of Education.

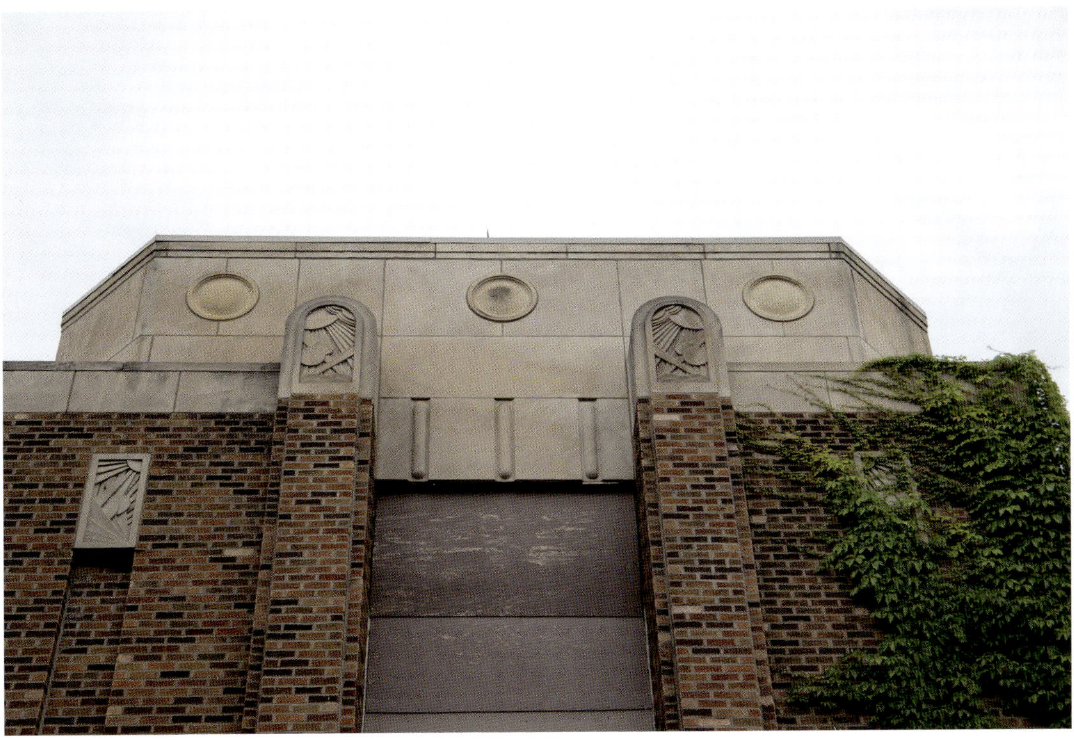

Beautiful architectural details.

Brown v. Board of Education

After Linda Brown was barred from attending Sumner, her father, Oliver Brown, and twelve other families filed a class-action lawsuit against the Board of Education of Topeka in 1952. At first, the plaintiffs lost and an appeal was filed and sent to the higher courts. They argued that segregation of public schools violated the "equal protection clause" of the 14th amendment, therefore no state could deny any person within its jurisdiction the equal protection of the laws. On May 17, 1954, Supreme Court justices unanimously voted that racial segregation in public schools was unconstitutional in the United States of America. This landmark decision would require schools across the country to desegregate, signifying the end of the "separate but equal" ruling put in place in 1896 by *Plessy v. Ferguson.*

Brown v. Board of Education II

Though the verdict was monumental, it did not specify how states should go about integrating their schools. Almost exactly one year later, the Supreme Court issued a second opinion, *Brown v. Board of Education II.* All future desegregation cases were remanded and sent to the district courts and school boards to continue with desegregation with deliberate speed. For Topeka, this resulted in multiple closing of schools and the opening of three more schools.

This caused a new problem. Now that the issue was in the hands of local officials, there was room for some evasion. Some states defied the *Brown v. Board* ruling. One of the most famous stories to come out of this defiance was when State National Guard troops were called in by Arkansas's governor to prevent the Little Rock Nine from entering Little Rock High School. This called for President Eisenhower to deploy federal troops to escort the nine students into the High School.

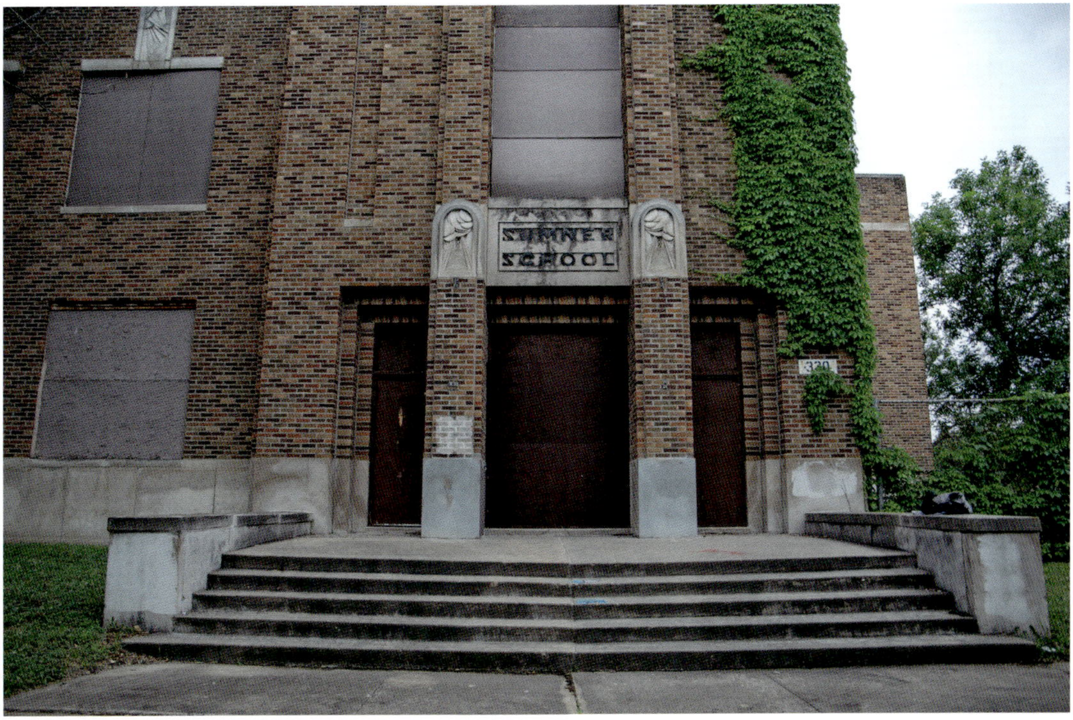

What elementary students would have seen walking into classes.

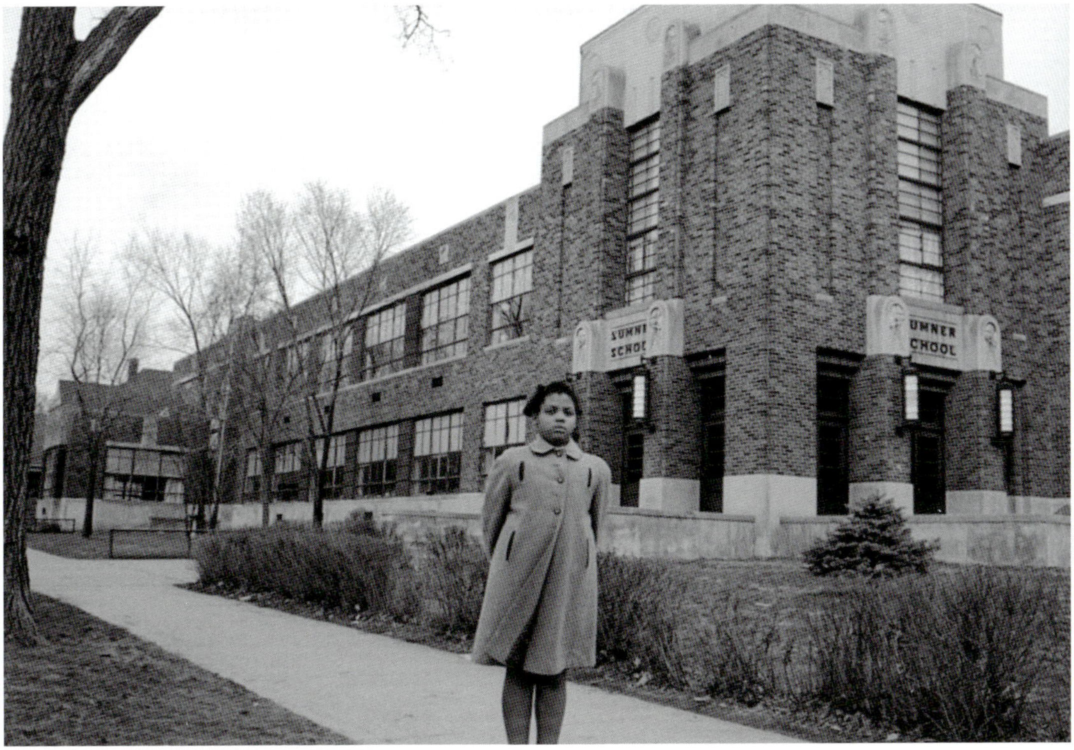

Linda Brown at nine, outside Sumner Elementary School in 1953 [*Carl Iwasaki, The LIFE Collection/Getty Images*]

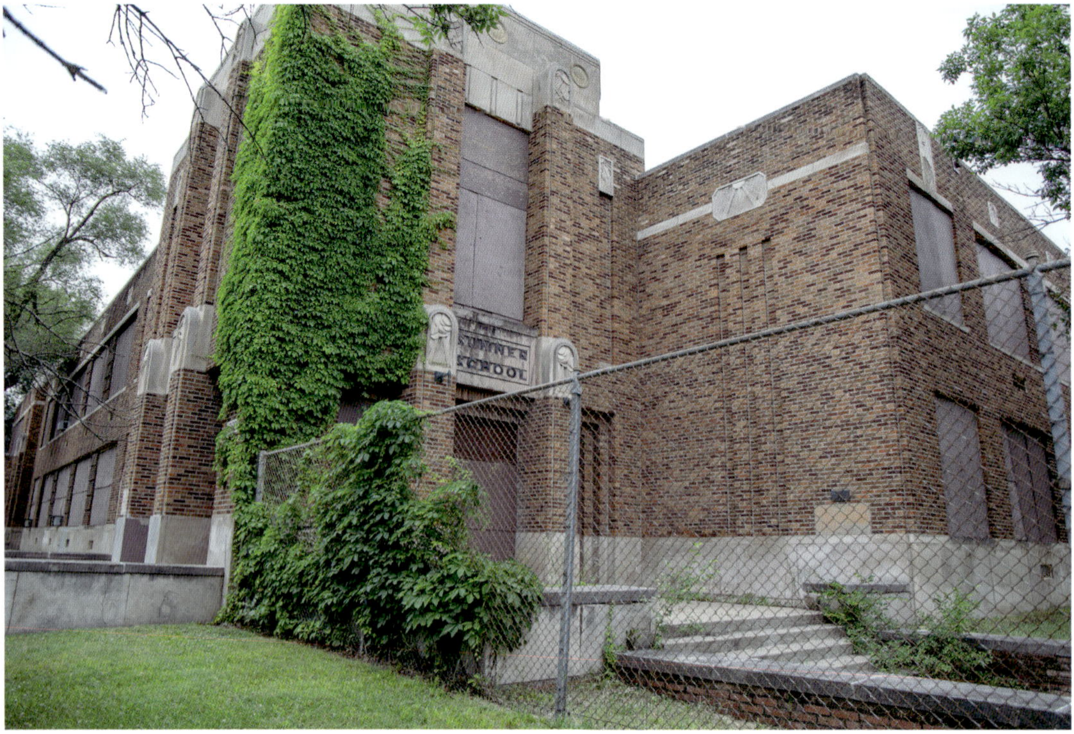

Nature attempts to reclaim the building.

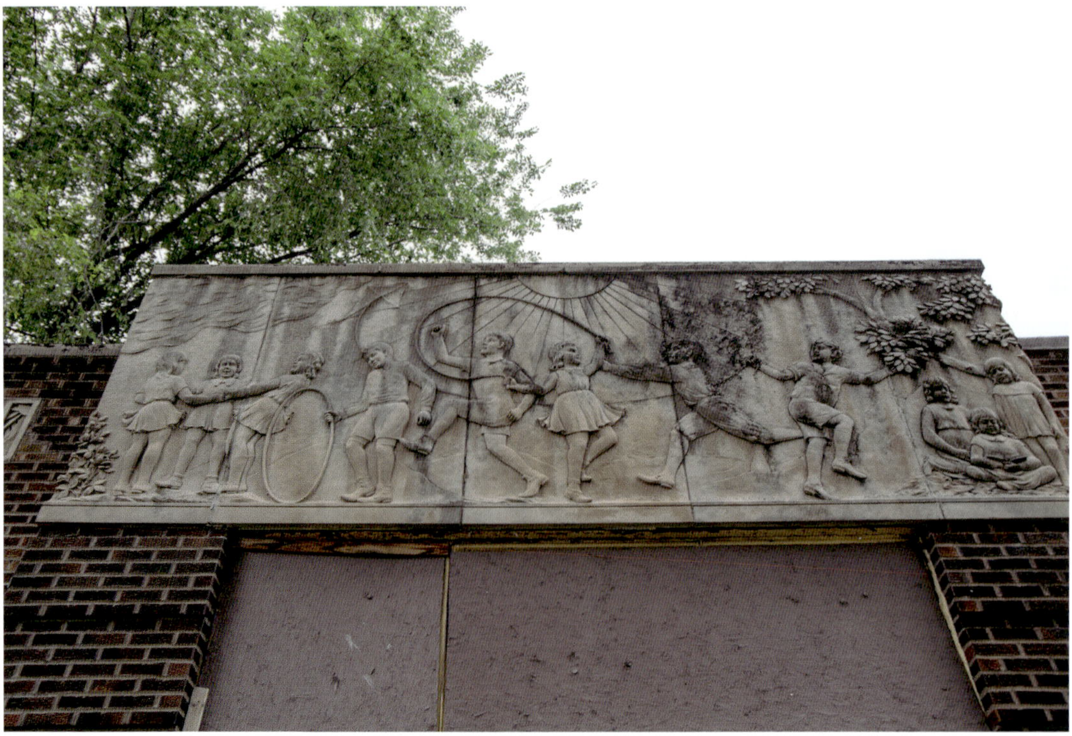

Intricate concrete mural next to kindergarten entrance.

Sumner Later Years/Closing

Tom Payne who attended from 1967-1972 said:

> Some of my best memories were at Sumner. In the summer, the school would provide a rec service for the neighborhood kids to come play games and they would provide us lunches. We had constant baseball games going on in the field. Some would last all day.
>
> We had Halloween parades where we got to go around the neighborhood and show off our costumes. Some years they were homemade, some years they were store bought. We had Christmas programs where each class prepared for several weeks to put on a skit or sing Christmas songs on stage in the auditorium in front of the other classes and parents.
>
> Since I lived so close to the school, only two doors down, at the end of the school year I would go over and help sort the school books out that were going to get replaced and the ones that were going to be used again the next school year.
>
> I had painful times there too. One summer day we were playing on the playground and a dog came onto the playground and started chasing us. He seemed playful so we didn't think much about it, but he ended up biting me, and since nobody knew whose dog it was or where he came from, I had to get rabies shots. Another time, we were playing baseball at recess. I was the catcher and the batter hit the ball, and after he hit it, he threw the bat and ran toward first, but when he threw, it hit me in the mouth, and I wasn't wearing a catcher's mask and had to get stitches. The guy that threw the bat was the best man at my wedding and I was the same at his. We still hang out together along with several of our friends from back then. My 4th-grade teacher from 1969 came to my dad's funeral service in 2007. That's how much of a family atmosphere there was.

On May 17, 1987, thirty-four years after the Supreme Court ruling, Sumner was honored as a National Historic Landmark by the U.S. Parks Service. A plaque was set on the building beside the front doors. It was later stolen in 2015. "I think it's a wonderful thing for the school to be declared a historic site. We waited many long years for the decision to be handed down," said Leola Brown-Montgomery, mother of Linda Brown, at the ceremony. Sumner was closed in 1996; it was one of eight Topeka schools closed as part of the original desegregation plan after the 1954 ruling. Shortly after the school was sold to the Topeka and Shawnee County Public Library and used as a storage facility. It was then purchased by the City of Topeka in 2002 with hopes to restore it, but they couldn't find the funds to do so. For the next couple of years attempts would be made to sell the building locally to no avail. The city even considered demolishing it after years of neglect and vandalism. *The Manhattan Mercury* reported on May 20, 2008, that the National

Trust for Historic Preservation had announced the school was named 1 of 11 most endangered places in America.

In October of 2008, it was decided by an 8-1 vote that the school be auctioned off with a required minimum bid of $50,000. It was sold to Southside Christian Palace Church of Los Angeles in April 2009 for $89,000. Archbishop W. R. Portee had the vision to restore Sumner to its once former glory and was in contact with BvB Legacy here in Topeka.

> Topekans have painfully watched Sumner deteriorate since Southside Christian Palace Church took ownership in 2009. The church did have good intentions, but no concrete plan for how to achieve them. They did let us—the Ward Meade neighborhood and Brown v. Board Sumner Legacy Trust (formed to help save Sumner)—help between 2012 and 2015, including cleanup inside the building and on the grounds during the 60th anniversary event in 2014 put together by locals. However, the church broke off that relationship in 2015. Since then, there has been further deterioration and no forward movement. Millions of dollars in renovation and interpretation grants and volunteer assistance have been missed. Further, various networks have emerged, all of which eagerly have reached out to BvBSLT (most with failed efforts engage the church as well) to include Sumner—the U.S. Civil Rights Trail, an emerging UNESCO World Heritage Site serial nomination for civil rights sites, a congressional request for a five-state partnership through the National Trust for Historic Preservation, the Crossroads of Freedom network through Freedom's Frontier National Heritage Area, the Kansas African American History Trail and Topeka's own growing Civil War to Civil Rights and heritage network.
>
> District 1's Councilwoman Karen Hiller

The Ward-Meade Neighborhood Association then sued the Southside Christian Palace Church in January of 2018 because the church had not followed through with their promise to restore the historic school. They are worried that the longer it sits, allowing for more destruction, the school's NRHP status could be endangered. The verdict was served in favor of Southside Church in January of 2019 on grounds that the deed does not specify a time frame in which the church has to restore Sumner. The Ward-Meade Neighborhood Association appealed, and the case is still going through the courts as of June 2021.

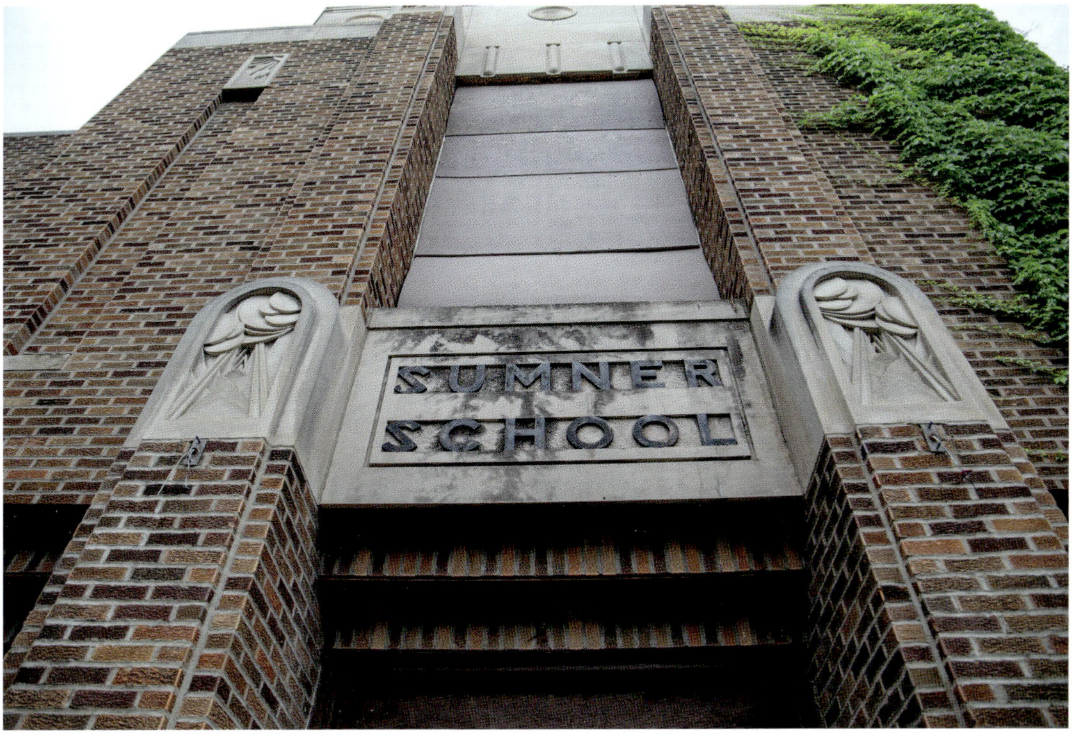

Sumner School entrance.

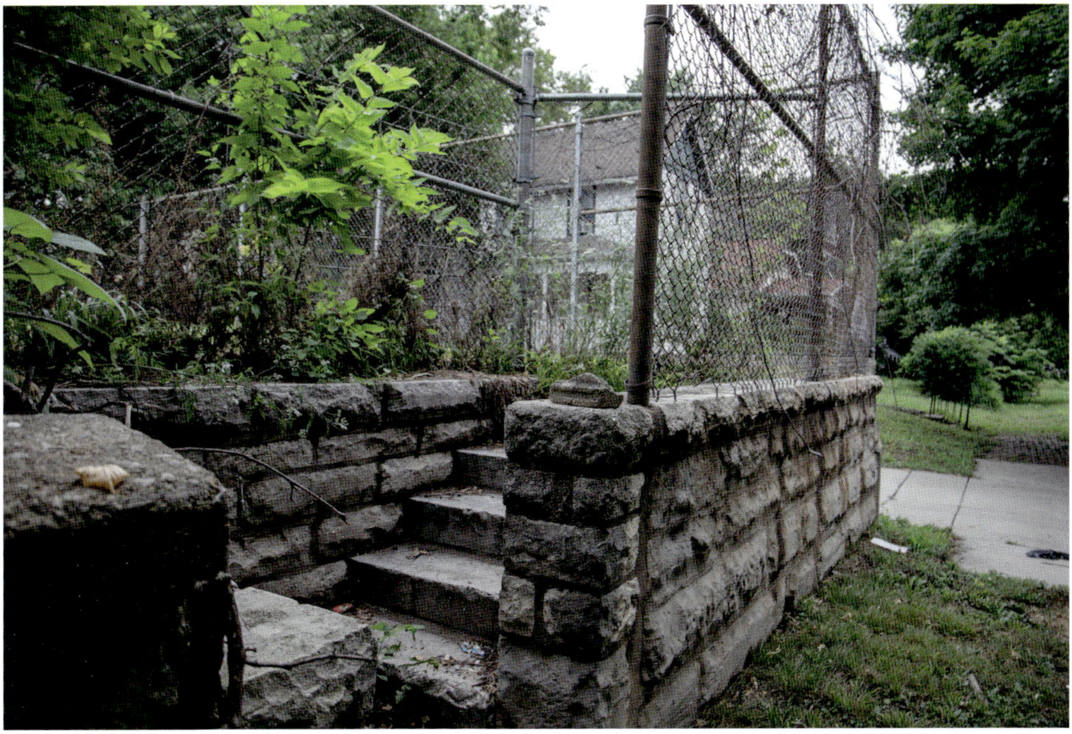

Steps into the playground area.

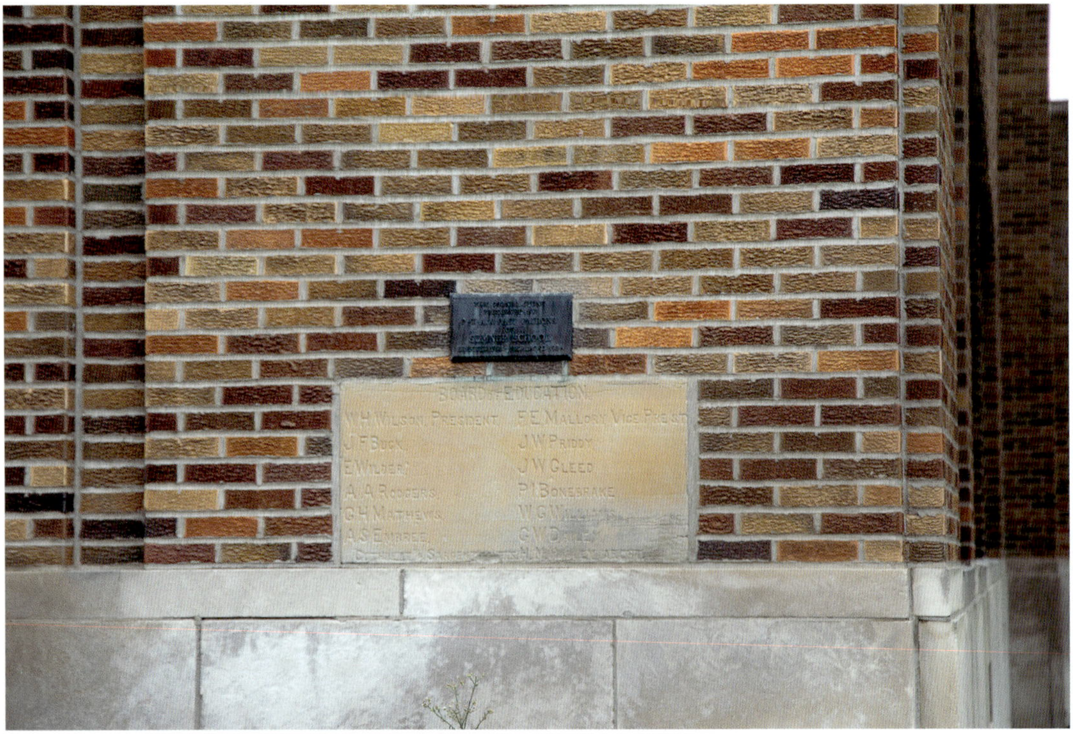

Cornerstone and replacement plaque of 1901 building.

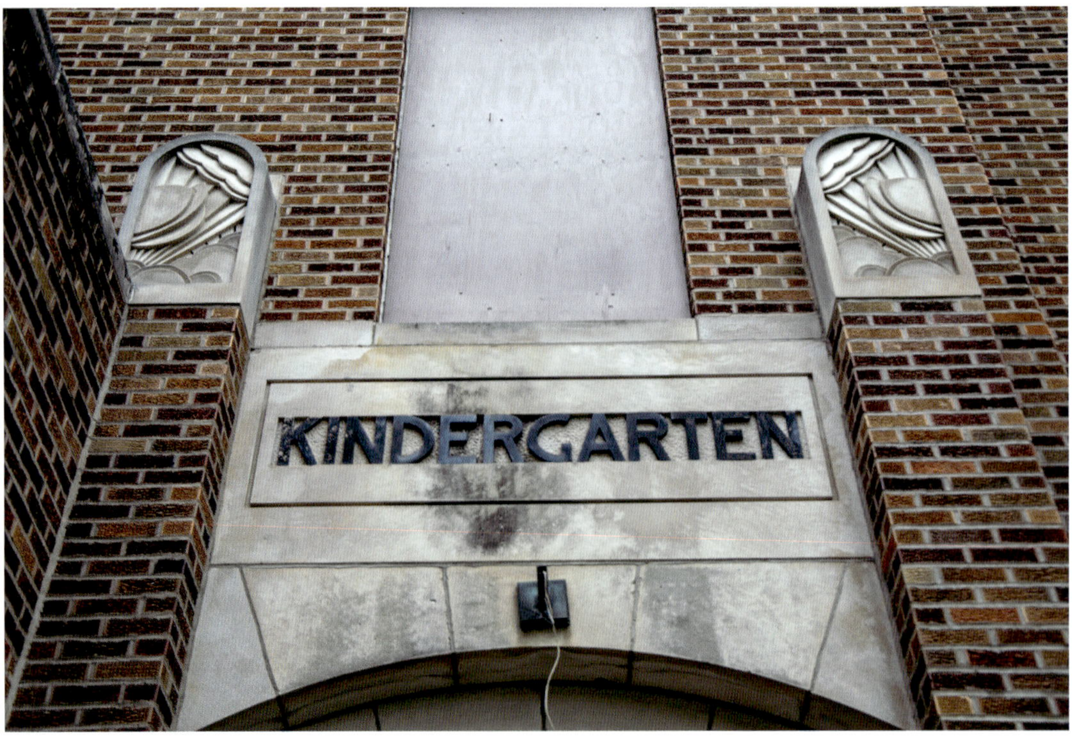

Kindergarten entrance.

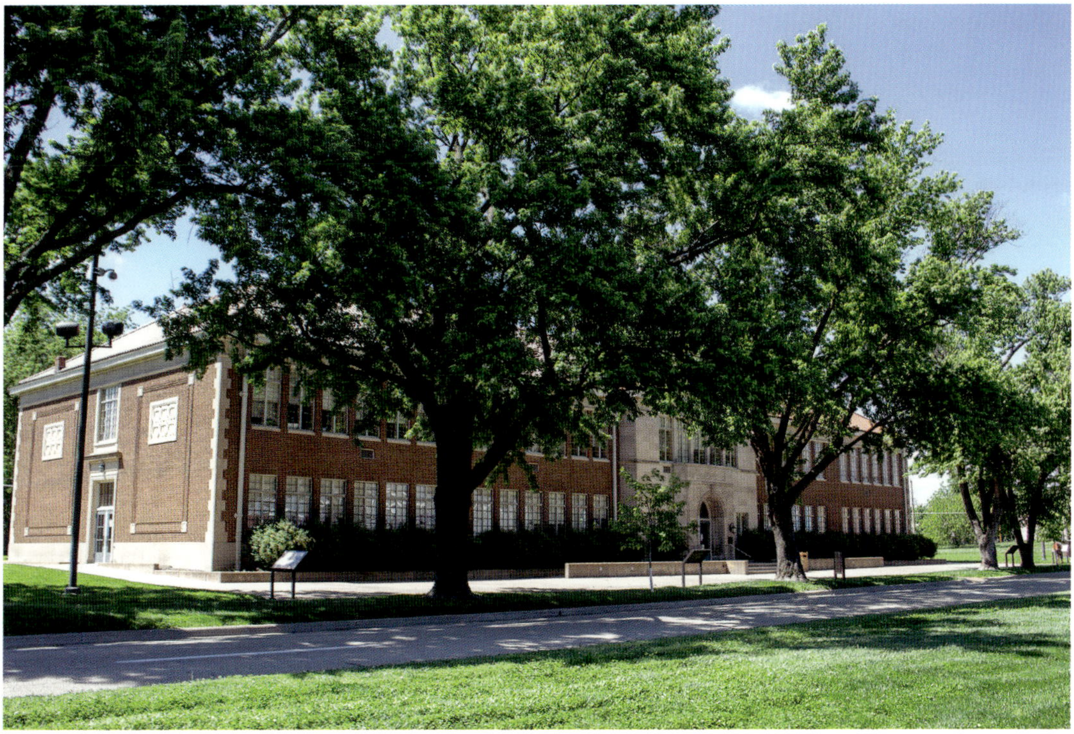

Above and below: Monroe School.

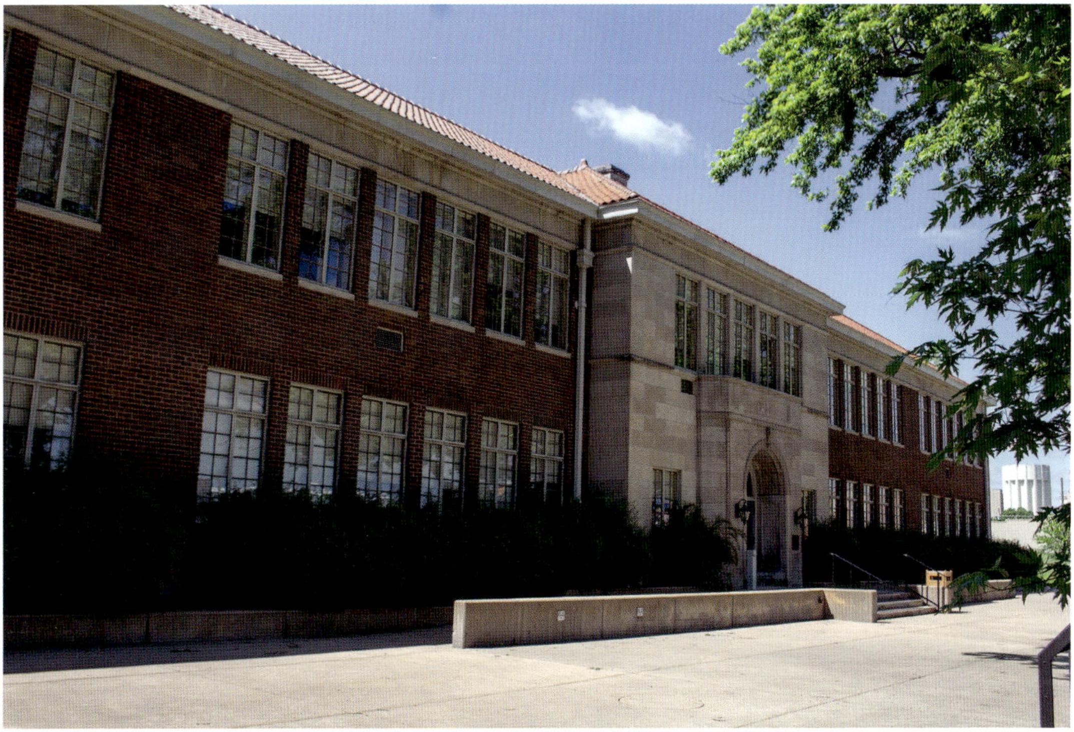

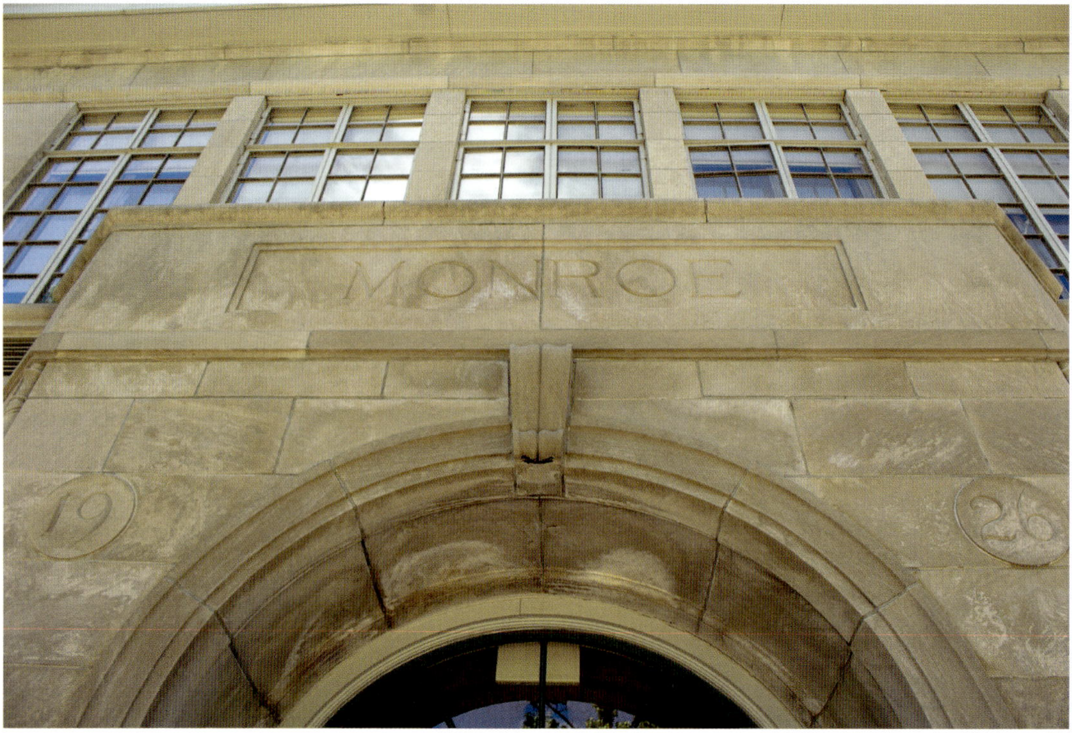

Engraving above the entrance.

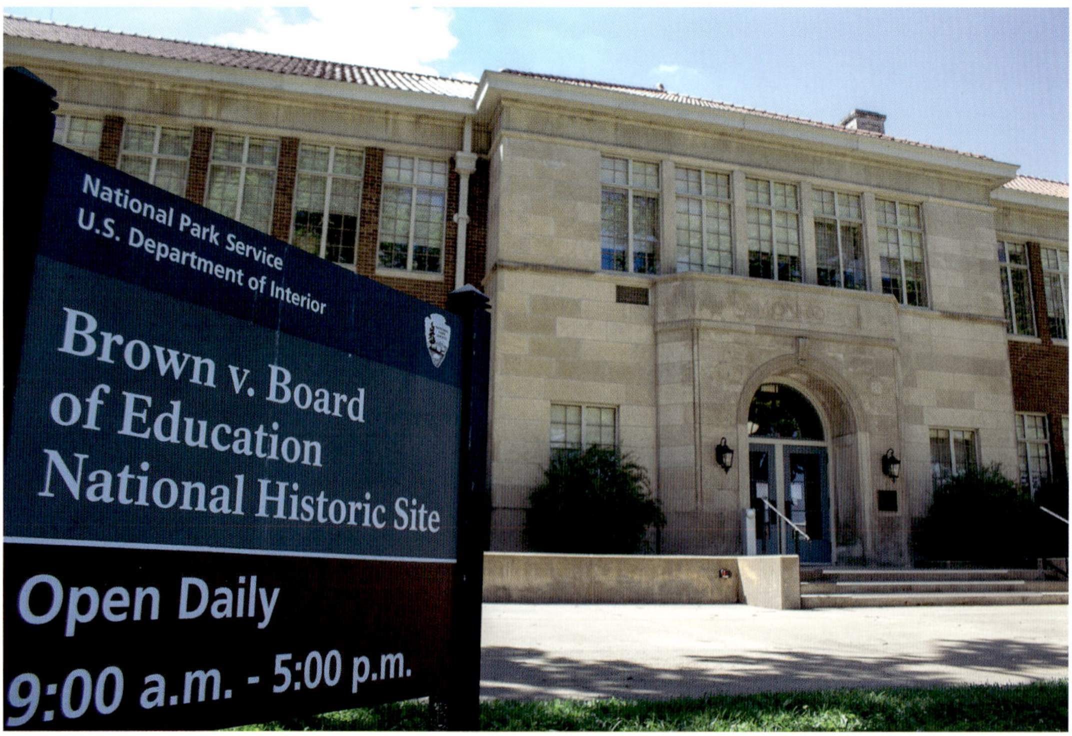

Brown v. Board of Education National Historic Site.

5

WHITE LAKES MALL

I had heard stories about this iconic Topeka shopping center when I was younger but didn't know that it had been closed since before I moved away. I grew up frequenting the West Ridge Mall. I remember going there to do my back-to-school shopping, getting a few items every year. I had no idea about the mall that my parents and family grew up going to and I was eager to find out.

A Real Hole-In-One

The land started out as the Topeka Golf Club, a pretty serious league that often challenged other nearby clubs, including the Kansas City Golf Club. The course attracted people from all over Topeka, and in 1933 the number of visitors grew.

In July of 1933, owner Joe White was enjoying the grand opening of his newly updated White Lakes Golf Club. The name was picked to highlight the three sparkling lakes at the course, infamous for sinking the balls of those whose aim was a bit off. The new club featured a renovated clubhouse with an updated kitchen, dining room, bar, locker/shower rooms, and pro shop. The new greens opened just in time for a two-day tournament. On December 23, 1947, the once public White Lakes Golf Club announced its plan to become a private club, thus becoming White Lakes Country Club.

In 1962, officials of the White Lakes Development Co. issued a statement to the public that a brand new $7-million shopping center would be built on the 35-acre property that used to be White Lakes Golf Club. It would be one of the first indoor, air-conditioned shopping centers in the Midwest, making it popular news amongst locals and those in the surrounding states. Ground was broken on February 6, 1963, by the White Lakes Development Co. and Keith Meyers. The final cost was $8 million, and the official opening day was October 15, 1964.

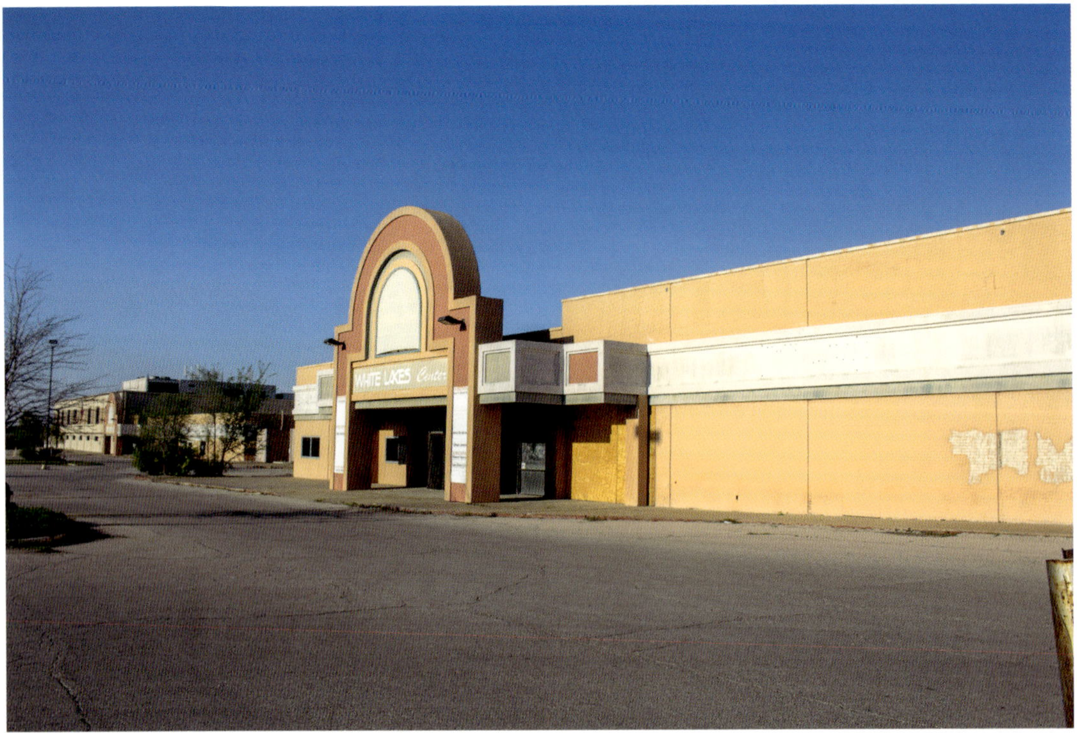

White Lakes Mall.

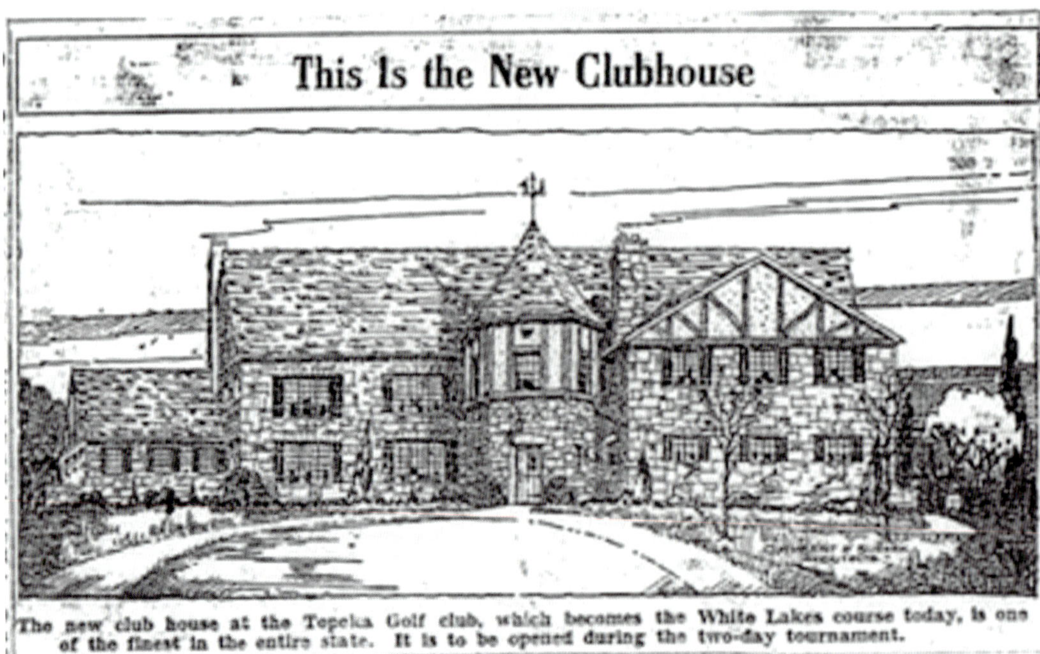
This Is the New Clubhouse

The new club house at the Topeka Golf club, which becomes the White Lakes course today, is one of the finest in the entire state. It is to be opened during the two-day tournament.

White Lakes Golf Clubhouse *ca.* 1933.

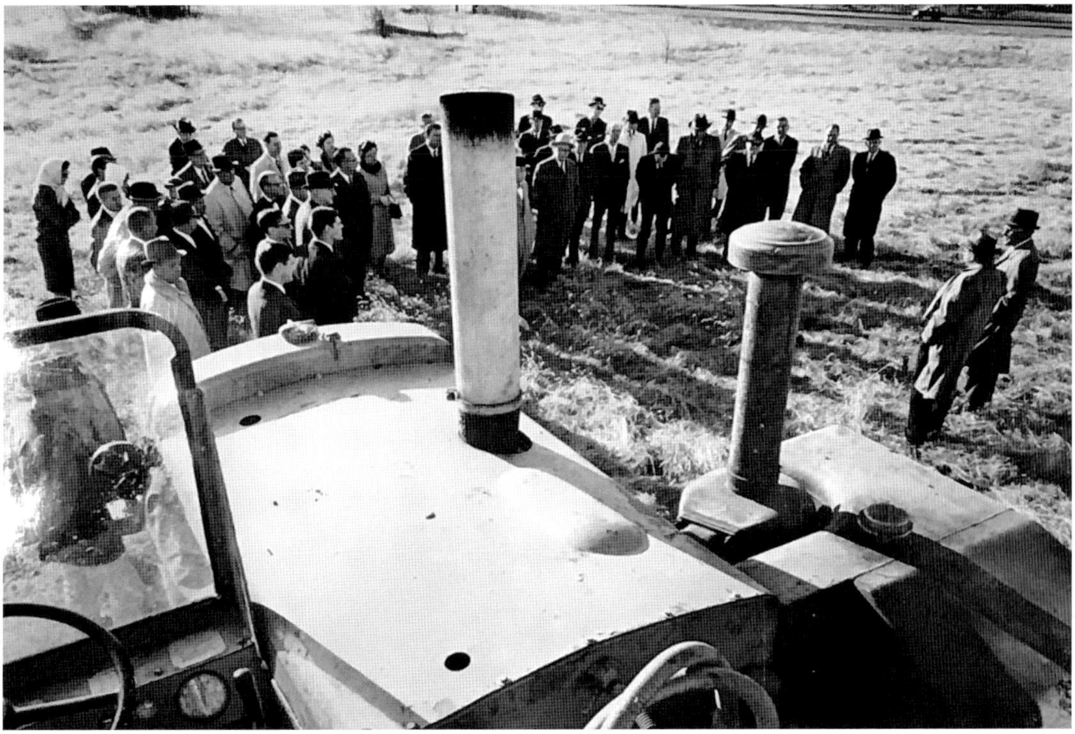

Groundbreaking of White Lakes Mall Feb 6, 1963. [*Susie Hoffmann*]

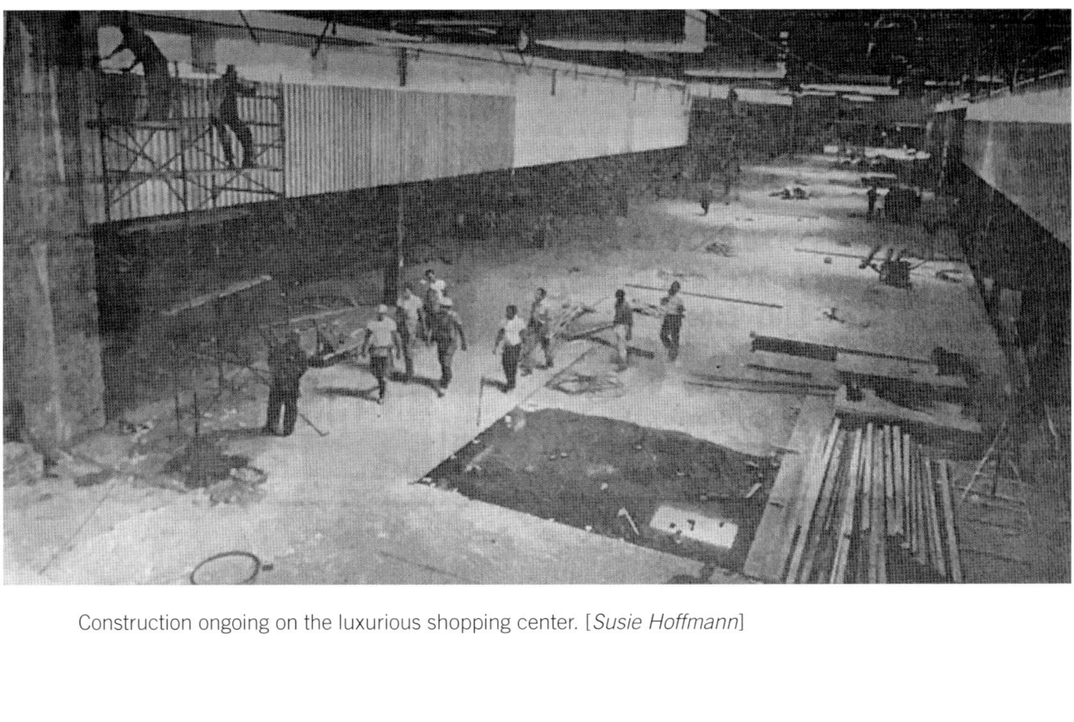

Construction ongoing on the luxurious shopping center. [*Susie Hoffmann*]

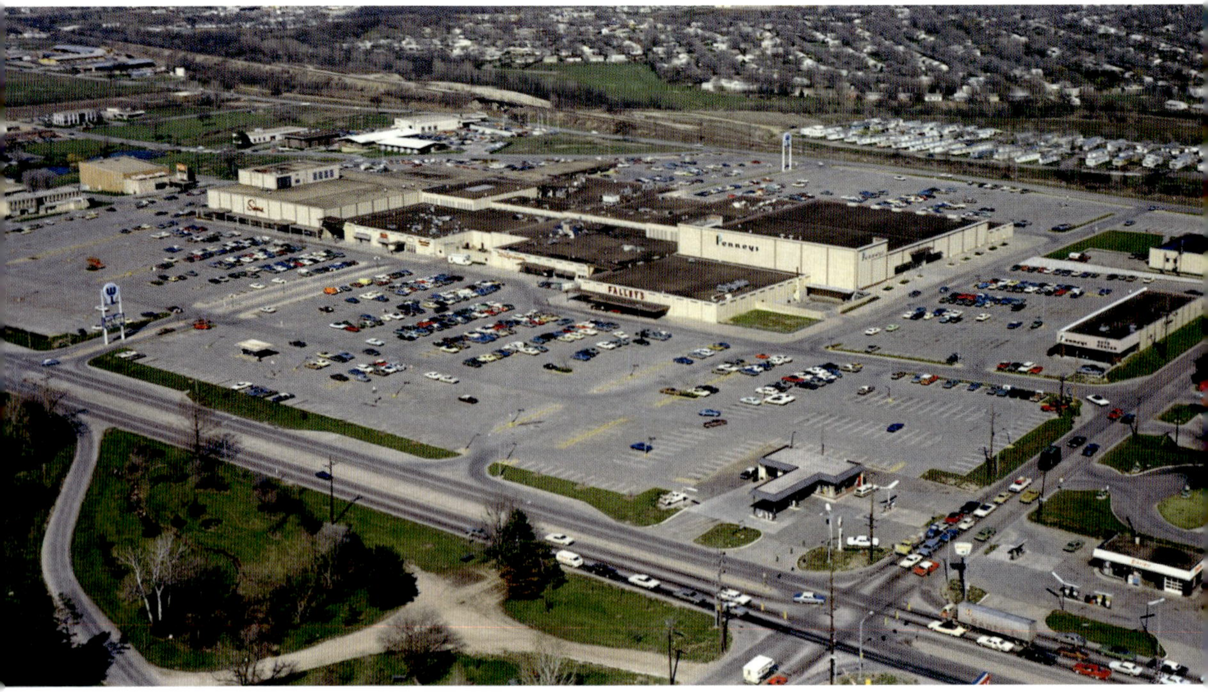

Aerial view of White Lakes Mall. [*Dave Mathias of Photo-1 Commercial Photography, 1973*]

Where Good Things Happen!

White Lakes Mall quickly gained two anchor stores: a two-story, 85,000-square-foot Sears on the north end, and a two-story, 52,300-square-foot J. C. Penney on the south end. The "new" J. C. Penney was the first full-line Penney store, including a freestanding auto center. Some other tenant stores there were Walgreens, Toy and Hobby Mart (which sold pets for a period of time), Command Performance Beauty Salon, Robinson's Shoes, and others. Falley's Market was a grocery store near the mall entrance doors that was accessible outside or from inside the mall. Having a grocery store within a mall was pivotal back then and relatively unheard of in a shopping center, even now. There were a few popular eateries in the shopping center as well. The Brass Rail was popular for their taco burgers, and the Town and Country Restaurant claimed to have the best onion soup and Swiss steak. The mall had unique features such as the cage which housed a squirrel monkey for a few years and then had live birds for a period of time after. There were also a few small koi ponds. One had a unique fountain flowing into it and was located by the cage, in front of J. C. Penneys. The other pond featured a small bridge over it and was in front of Sears. This area would also be set up with a stage for the Marionette Puppet Shows during the Christmas season. It coined the slogans "Where the Good Things Happen!" and "It's Always a Comfortable 72 Degrees at White Lakes Mall!"

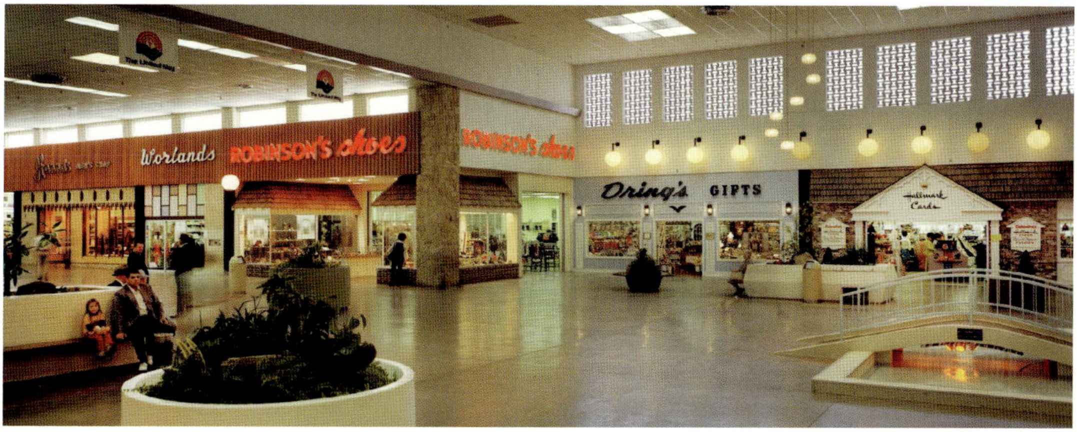

White Lakes Mall during Christmas time. [*Dave Mathias of Photo-1 Commercial Photography, 1972*]

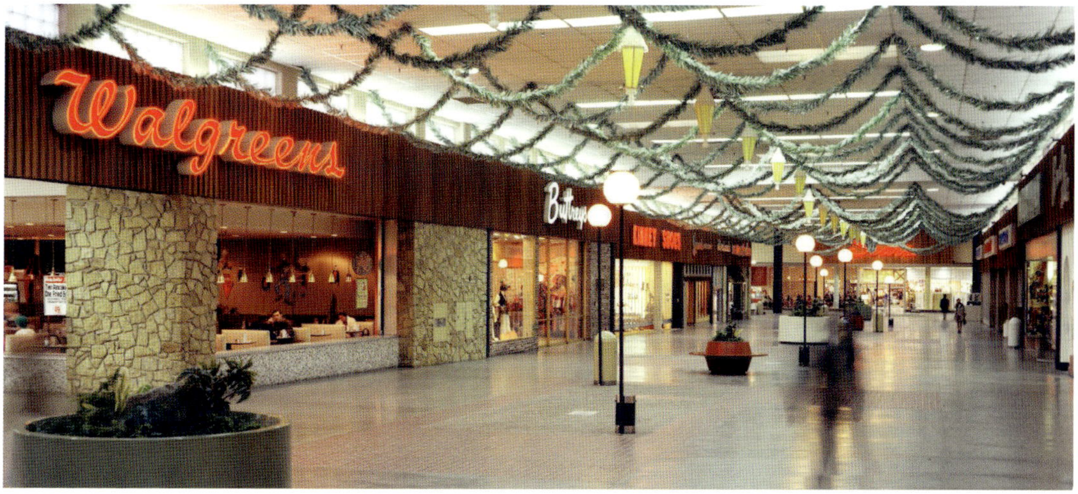

Strip of shops around Christmas time in White Lakes. [*Dave Mathias of Photo-1 Commercial Photography, 1972*]

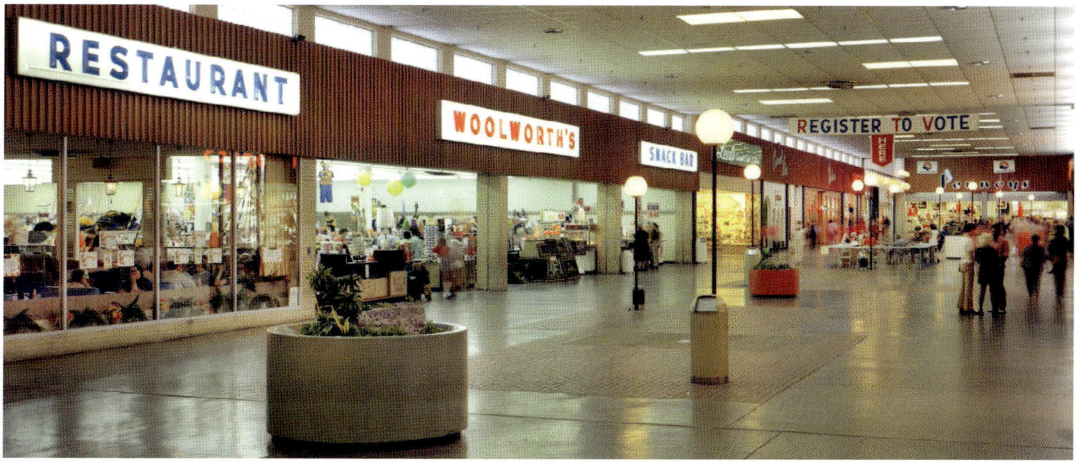

White Lakes Mall during Christmas time. [*Dave Mathias of Photo-1 Commercial Photography, 1972*]

I grew up at White Lakes. My family owned The Hat Box and The Hat Box II. We were the "boutique" that pierced ears, located next to The Brass Rail down by Sears. My grandma, Helen Gish, started the business. She was an original tenant when the mall opened. Her brother, Keith Meyers, was the developer and part owner of the mall and her brother-in-law, Tom Martin, owned the construction company that built the mall. My mom started working in the business after I was born. I worked there during junior high, high school and college. For ten years, three generations of us Gish/Hoffmann's worked at the shop. I ate many tacos from The Brass Rail and lots of patty melts from Sears. I have such fond memories of the mall. I took sewing lessons from the Singer sewing/fabric store and candy making classes upstairs at J. C. Penneys. Many years ago, when they remodeled the mall and took out the bridge over the koi pond down by Sears, my grandma bought the bridge handrails. My grandpa built a bridge in their backyard with the handrails. I have since bought my grandparents' home and just this summer rebuilt the bridge. There were layers and layers of baby blue paint under the black paint my grandpa had painted.

Susie Hoffmann

The shopping mall's demise came slowly and painfully with the attention turned to the brand-new mall opening up on the West side of town. In 1988, the 992,000-square-foot West Ridge Mall had opened, making it almost twice the size of the 500,000-square-foot White Lakes Mall. By the time of its grand opening, it had already snatched up the two anchor stores, Sears and J. C. Penneys, of White Lakes. With the elimination of both anchor stores in the mall, other tenants followed in hopes of gaining more business, since people were flocking to the new and updated mall of West Ridge. Housing developments sprung up to the west of the city, closer to the new mall. Eventually, remaining businesses at White Lakes were faced with the choice to shut down or move closer to "the action."

Growing up it was a special treat to get to go to Topeka and "the mall" which meant White Lakes until the late 80s, when West Ridge came in. I loved White lakes. I miss the familiarity and simplicity; it's been there as long as I can remember. My husband and I's love story began at White Lakes on a freezing January 22, 1983. Topeka Blvd. was where everyone went cruising and the mall was where everyone hung out on the weekends. I was with a couple friends sitting in the parking lot when my husband, Bert, and a couple of his friends, who were actually supposed to be meeting some friends there, accidentally thought our vehicle was their friends'. They pulled in next to us and we started talking, went on a date the next weekend, *and here we are still together* thirty-seven years later. In the late 80s/ early 90s, we lived on SW Kerry Ave. across the street from White Lakes and could see it from our home as it became an eyesore.

Patty Lanum about the Center

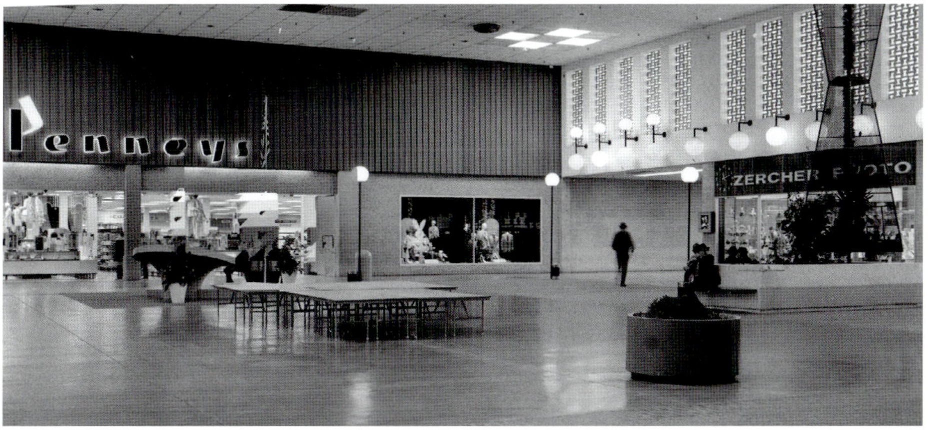

Penneys, now known as J. C. Penneys, located in the South hub. [*Dave Mathias of Photo-1 Commercial Photography, 1973*]

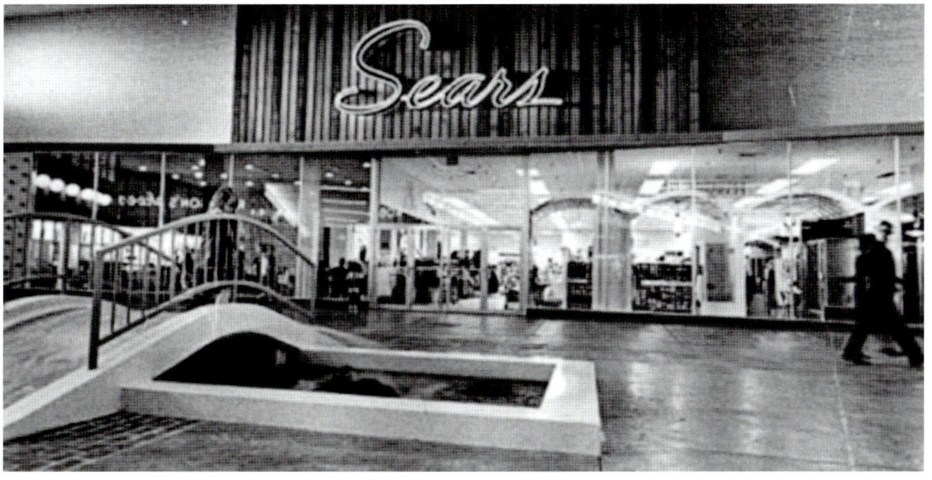

Water feature bridge in front of Sears in the North hub. [*Dave Mathias of Photo-1 Commercial Photography, 1973*]

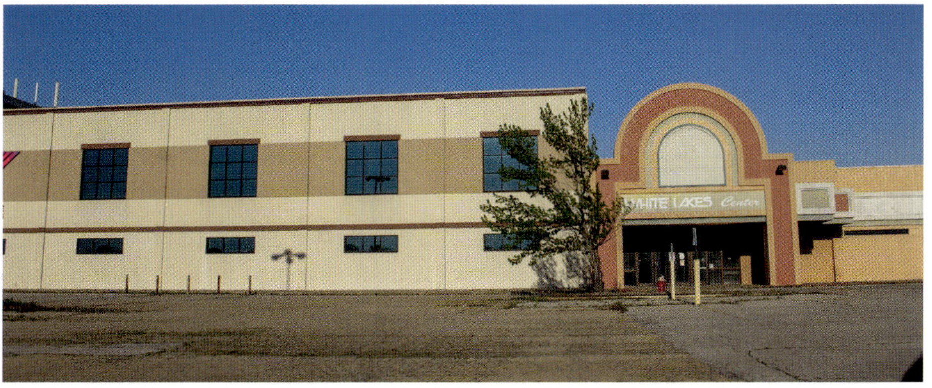

Mainline Printing inhabits the old Sears store. Only a wall separates the inhabited business from the neglected mall.

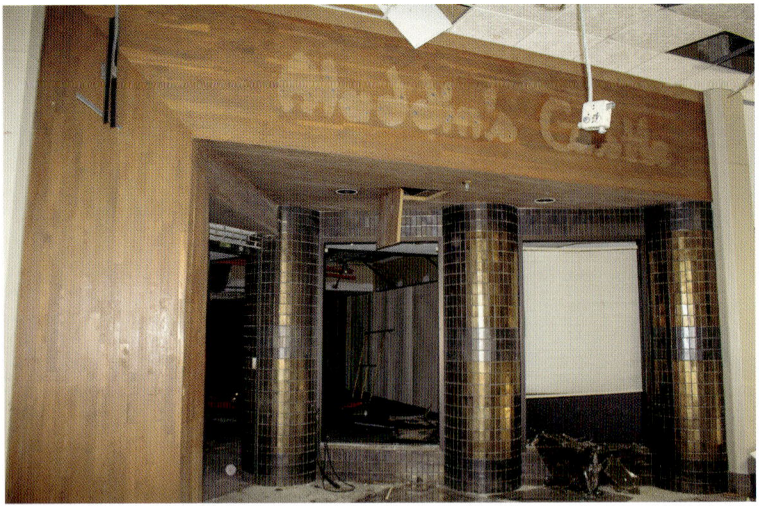

Aladdin's Castle Arcade.

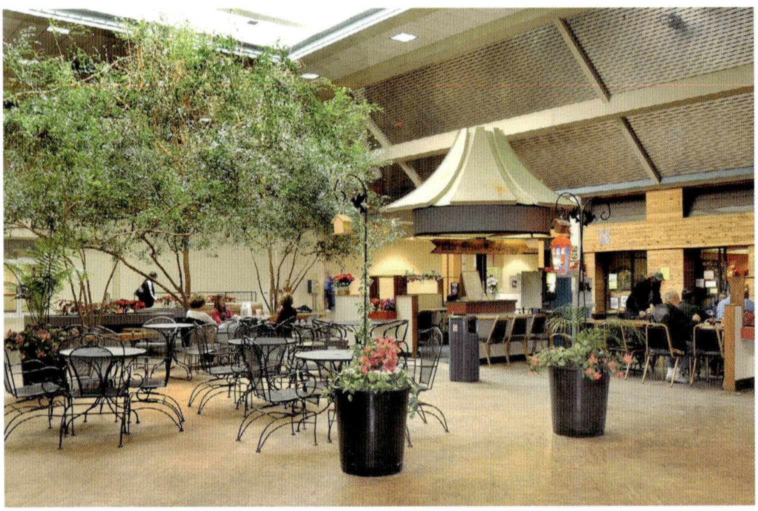

At a later date, the Orange Julius stand became a different shop. [*Dave Mathias of Photo-1 Commercial Photography, 2008*]

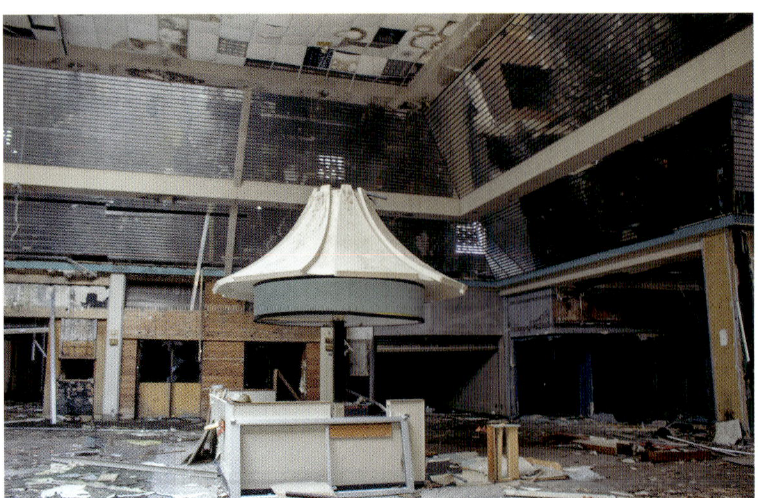

Former Orange Julius stand.

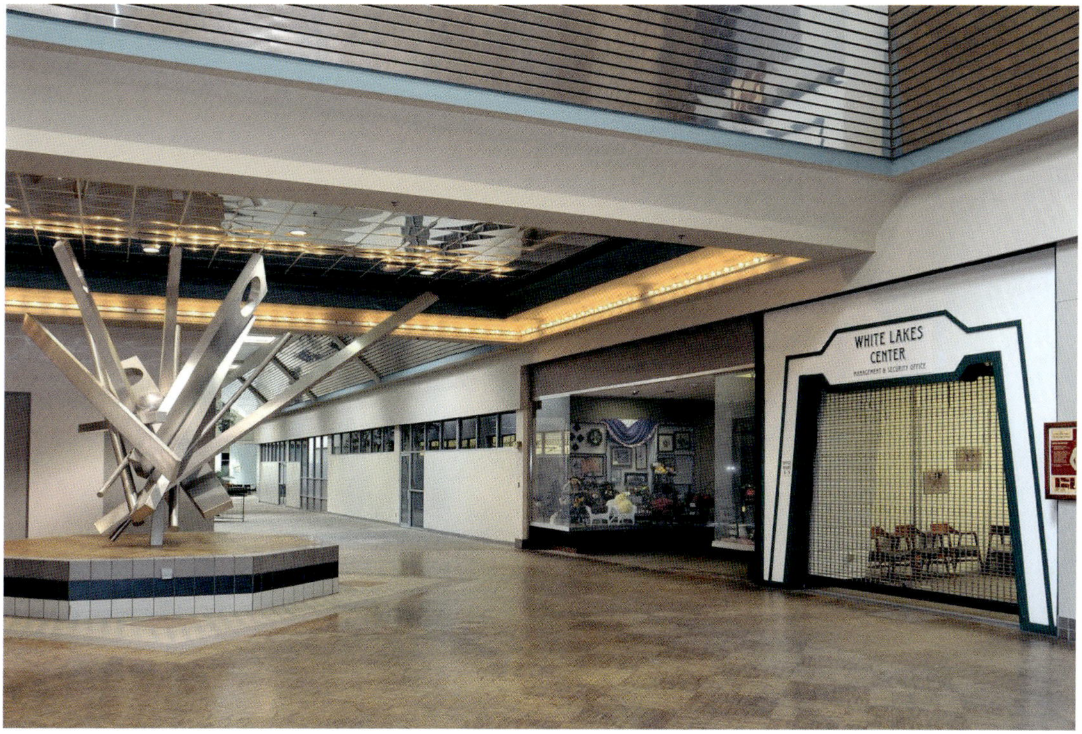

This sculpture was moved in 2012 and is now located at 921 S.W. Topeka Blvd. [*Dave Mathias of Photo-1 Commercial Photography, 2008*]

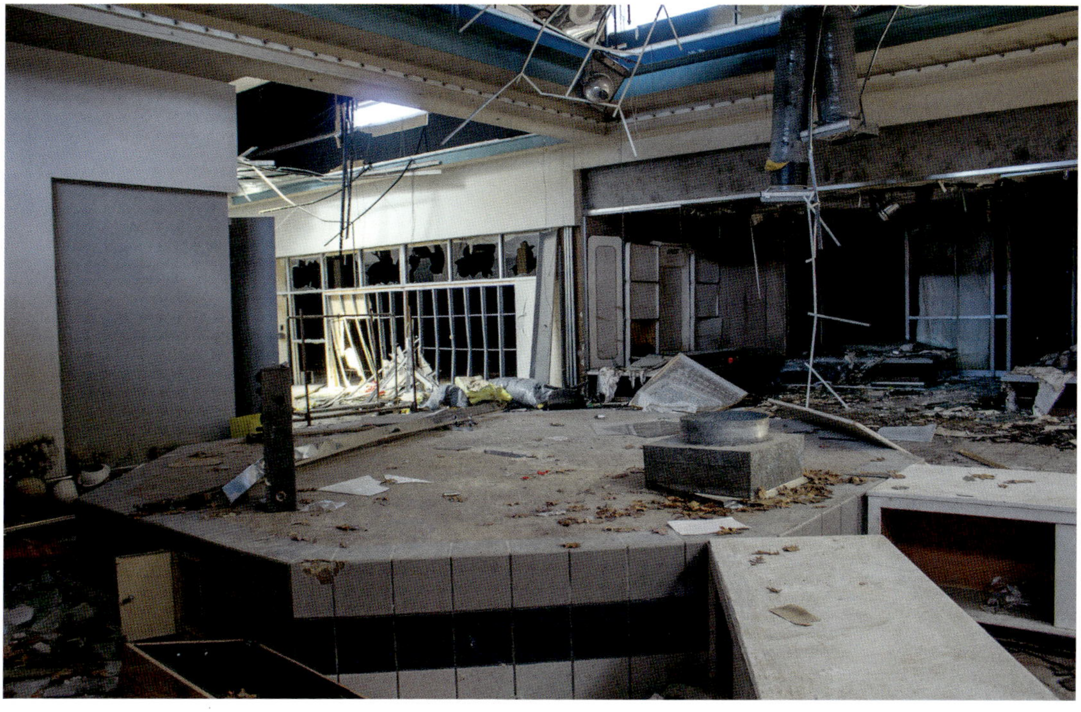

Stage where the sculpture used to stand.

The End of an Era

By 2000, most of the stores had either gone out of business or moved elsewhere, and the shopping mall was converted into an office complex with a few retail and service stores left. It was renamed White Lakes Center, keeping ties to its roots. Tenants included Walgreen Drug that had been in the mall since opening, Electronic Data Systems, Blue Cross & Blue Shield, Kansas Children's Services League, the State of Kansas, Kansas Rehabilitation, a daycare center, fitness center, beauty salon, and several restaurants. Mainline Printing moved into the old Sears portion of the building in 2004, renovating 190,000 square feet of it.

Around 2007, a large majority of companies that used the office spaces moved out, resulting in many vacancies. The building was put up for sale; it sold to Kent Lindemuth on September 30, 2009. Lindemuth's plans started with wanting to divide the former mall into two or three buildings offering the same amenities but in a different vision. Instead of being connected by the inside mall walkway, he wanted to demolish it and create a new vision of exterior-entranced retail and office space. The few tenants that remained from the previous ownership started receiving eviction notices and those that hadn't were waiting to look for a new place to relocate.

Mr. Lindemuth, unfortunately, filed for bankruptcy in November 2012 and was found to be around $45 million in debt. He was a veteran businessman and investor within the city and his bankruptcy caused reverberations to crash through the Topeka business community. This was before the new White Lakes renovations could take place and the once popular Topeka landmark became abandoned. The only business that has remained at the site is Mainline Printing, who resides in the portion of the mall that used to be home to Sears. They have secluded themselves from the rest of the neglected portion of the mall by putting up a secure wall between themselves and the abandonment. But this hasn't fully protected the company from the dangers that the neglected mall has brought. At around 6:30 a.m. on December 29, 2020, the Topeka Fire Department received calls about a blaze protruding through the rough of the derelict White Lakes Mall. A giant fire was eating its way through the building and pouring out of the roof. Because of the deterioration, asbestos, and black mold present in the building, firefighters were not able to enter the building. Flames were fought by firefighters on ladders extended over the roof, pouring gallons of water in an attempt to keep the fire from reaching the Mainline Printing business. It was first speculated that it was an accidental fire started by one of the many squatters that called the building home, but it was discovered a few days later that it was intentionally set. Three teenagers were arrested on charges of arson, criminal damage to property, and criminal trespassing for causing the $100,000 worth of damage to White Lakes Center.

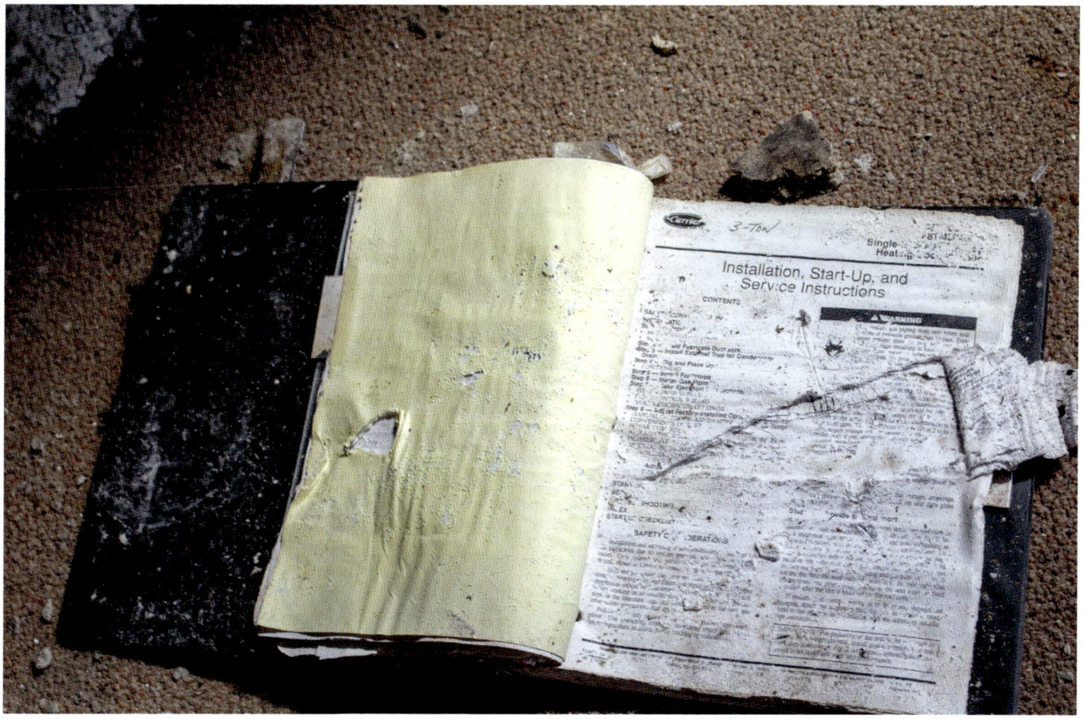

Installation, Start-Up & Services manual.

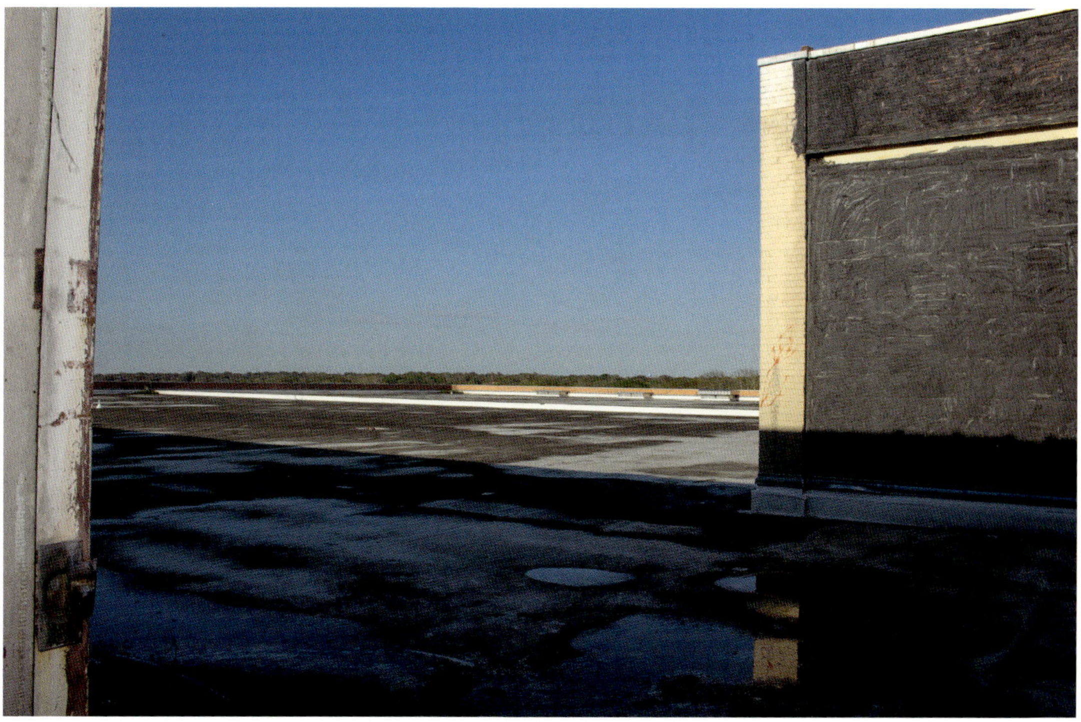

Rooftop view.

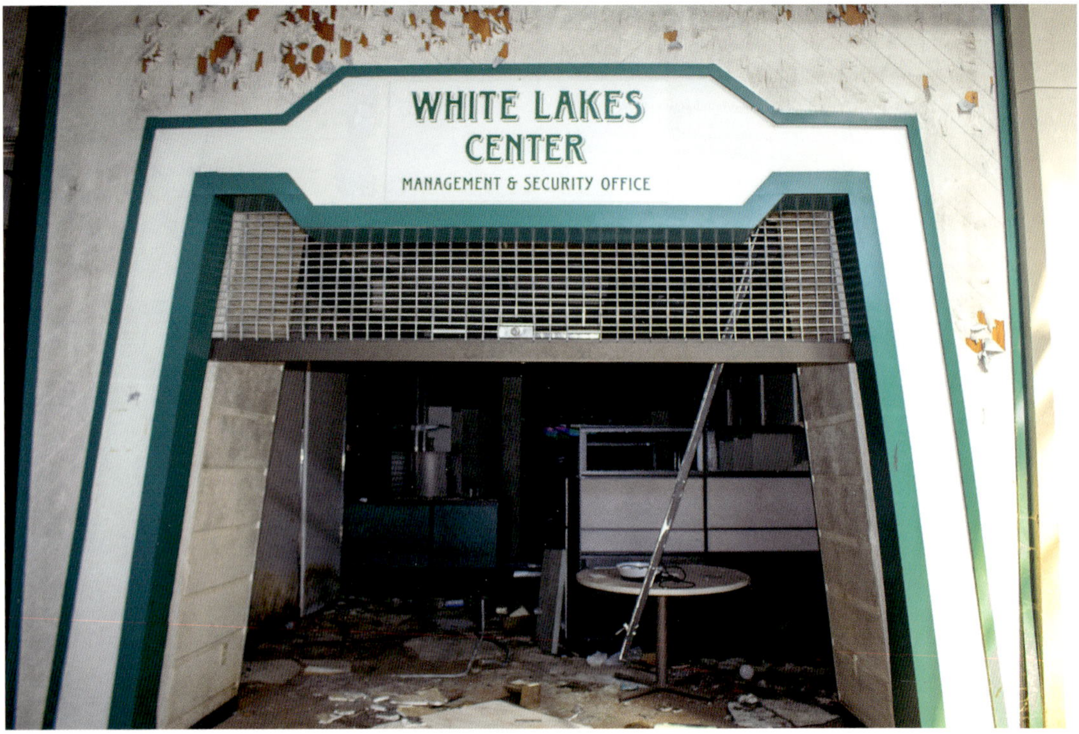

Above and below: White Lakes Center Management & Security Services office.

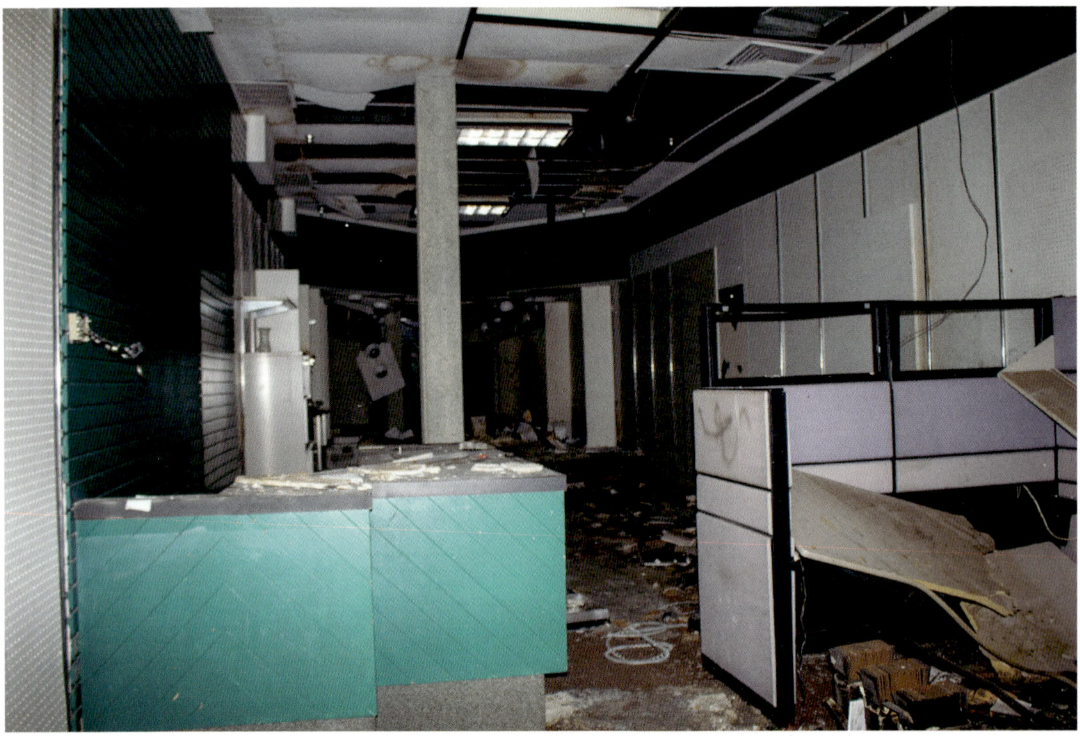

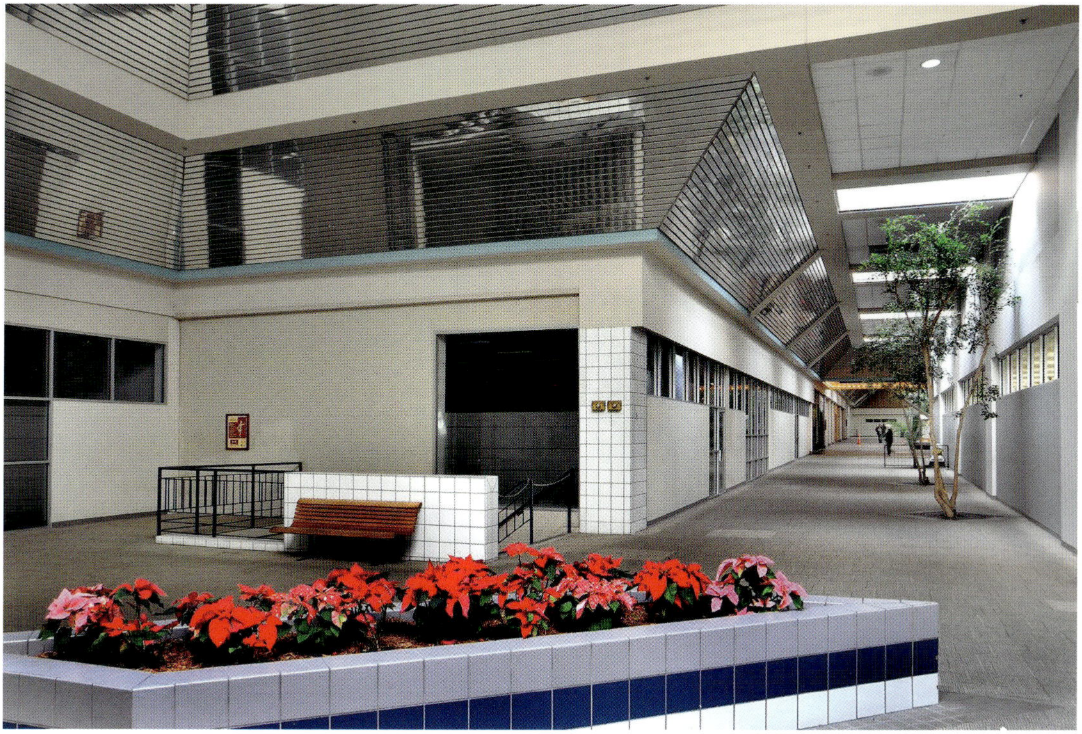

Hallway to the North hub. [*Dave Mathias of Photo-1 Commercial Photography, 2008*]

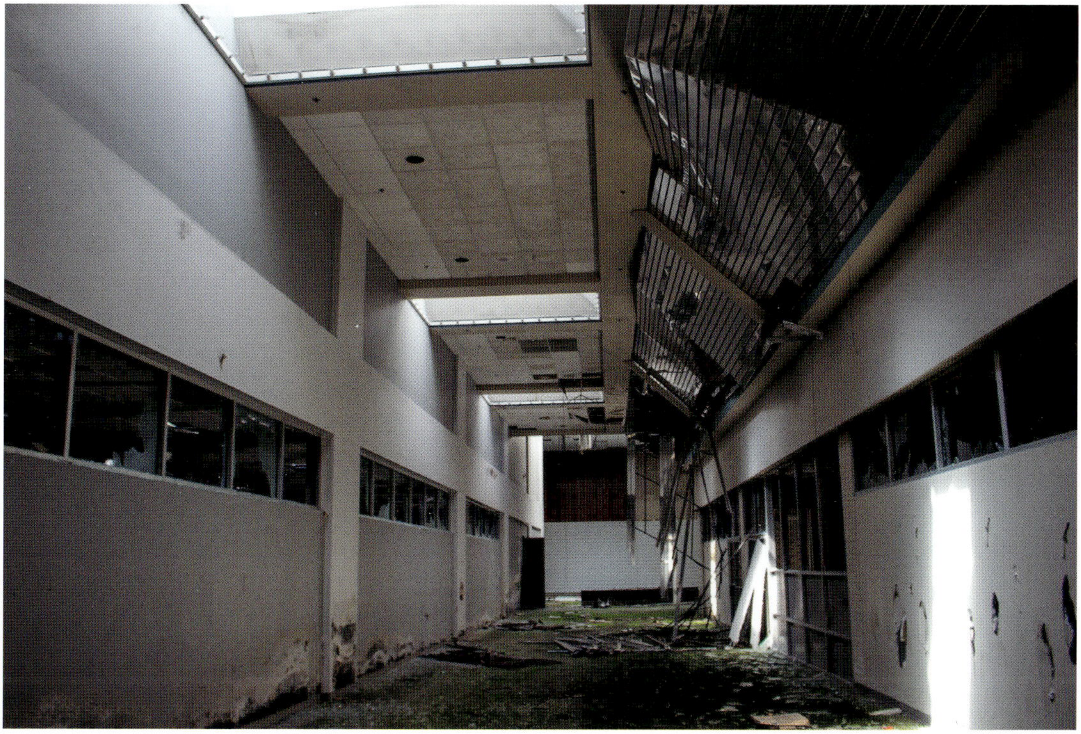

Hallway to the North hub.

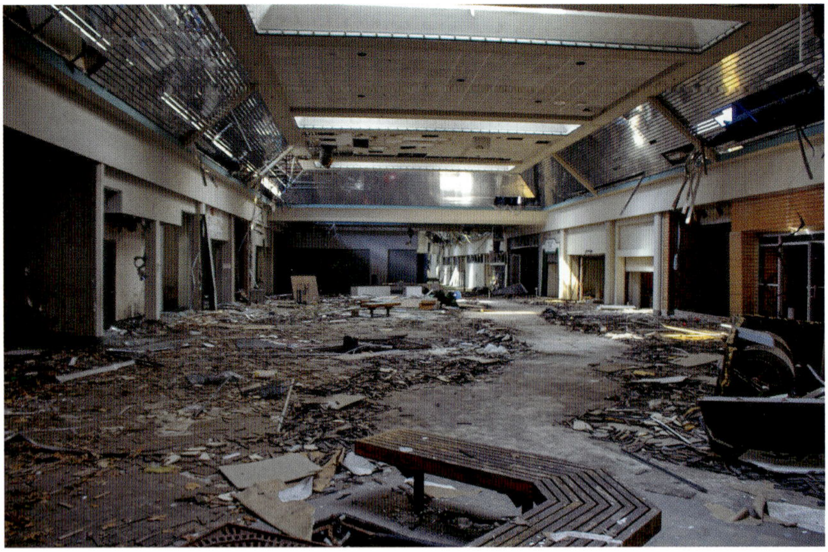

Walk down memory lane.

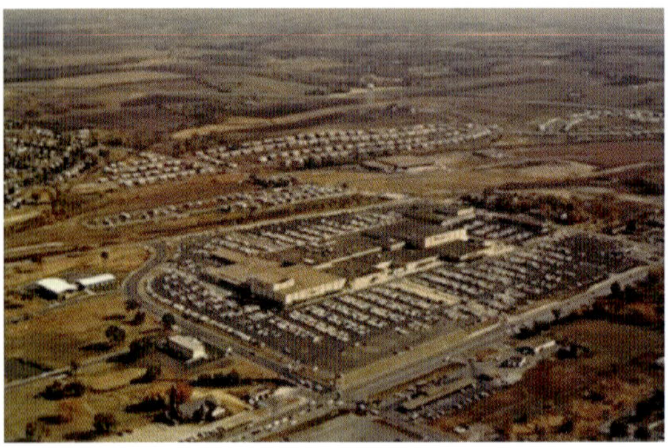

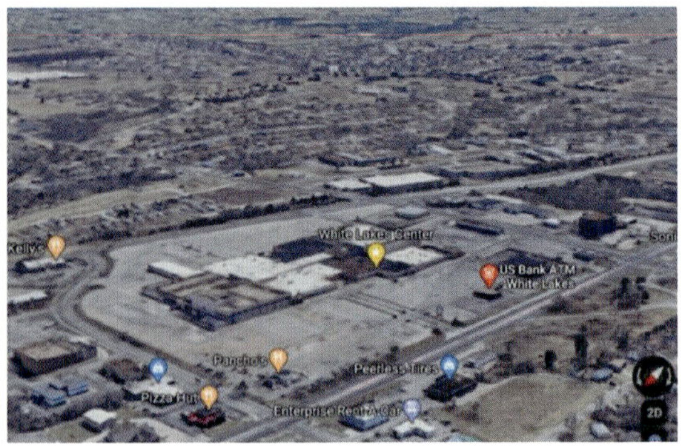
White Lakes Center
US Bank ATM
White Lakes
Pizza Hut
2D

1960s left vs. 2021 right, comparison of White Lakes Mall.

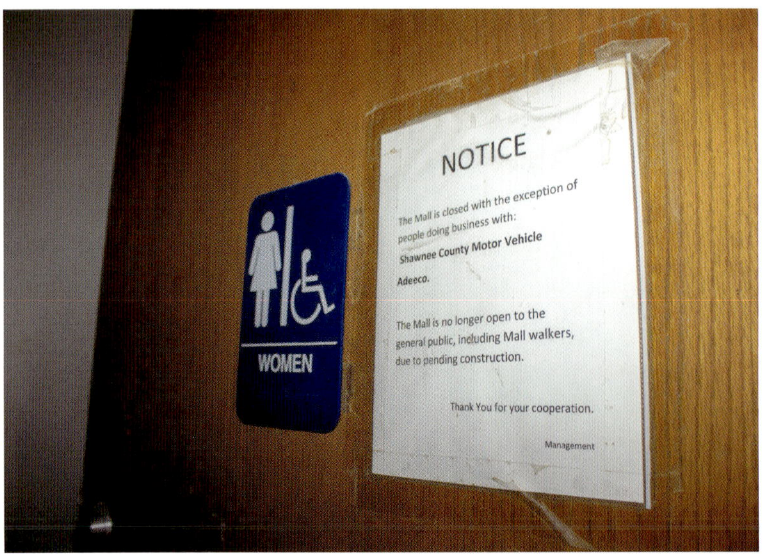
WOMEN
NOTICE
The Mall is closed with the exception of people doing business with:
Shawnee County Motor Vehicle
Adeeco.
The Mall is no longer open to the general public, including Mall walkers, due to pending construction.
Thank You for your cooperation.
Management

Notice of the White Lakes Centers' closure.

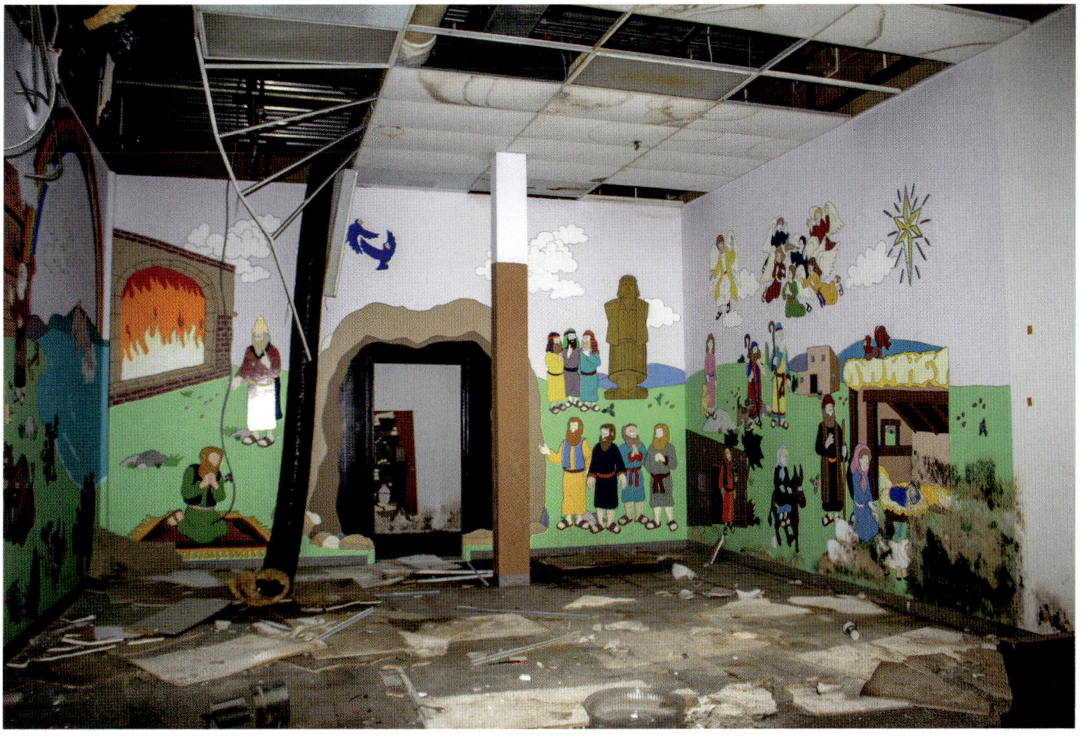

Holy Grounds Coffee Shop.

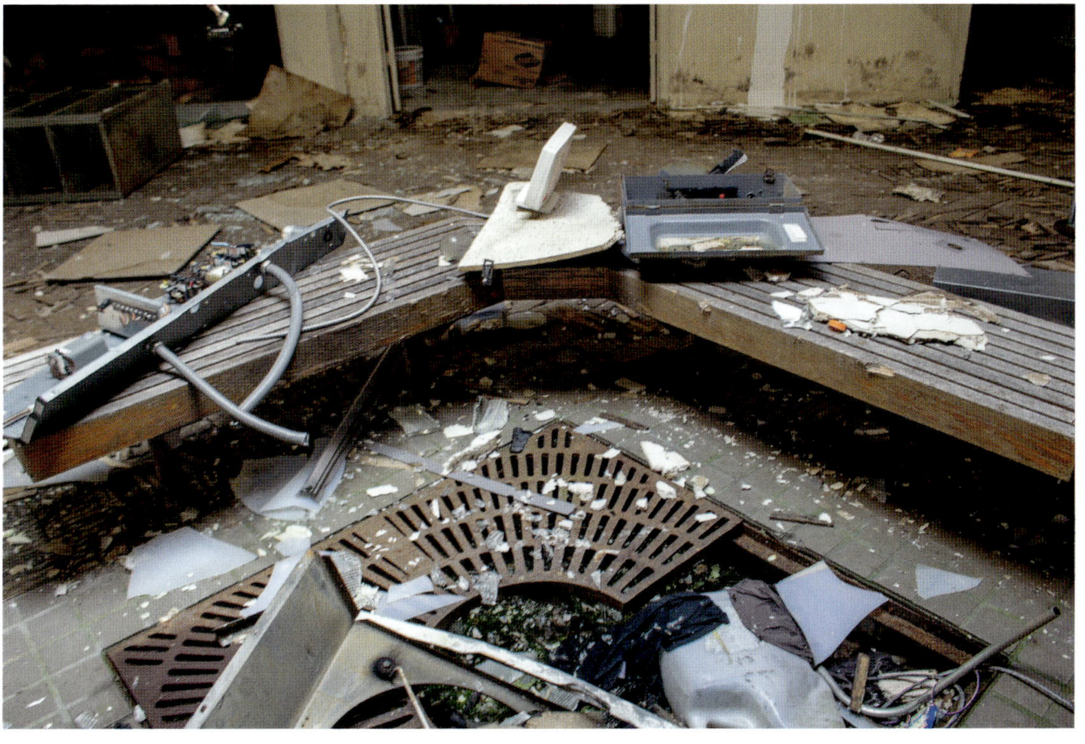

Grates where a tree used to stand with a bench next to it.

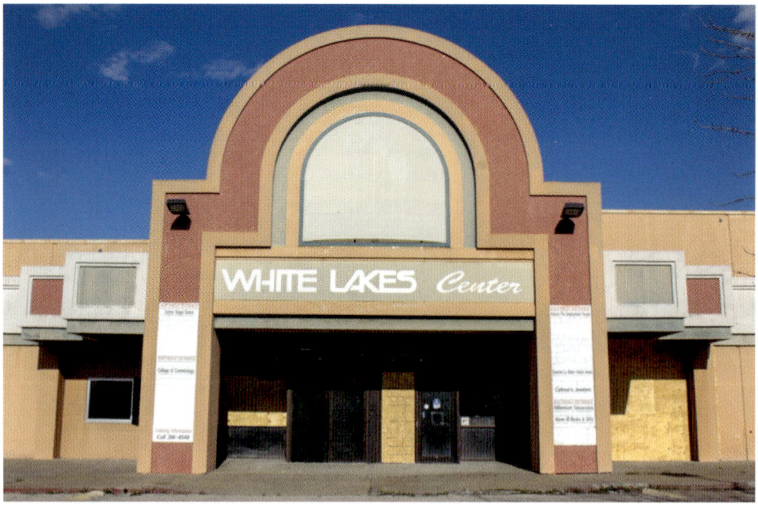

White Lakes Center.

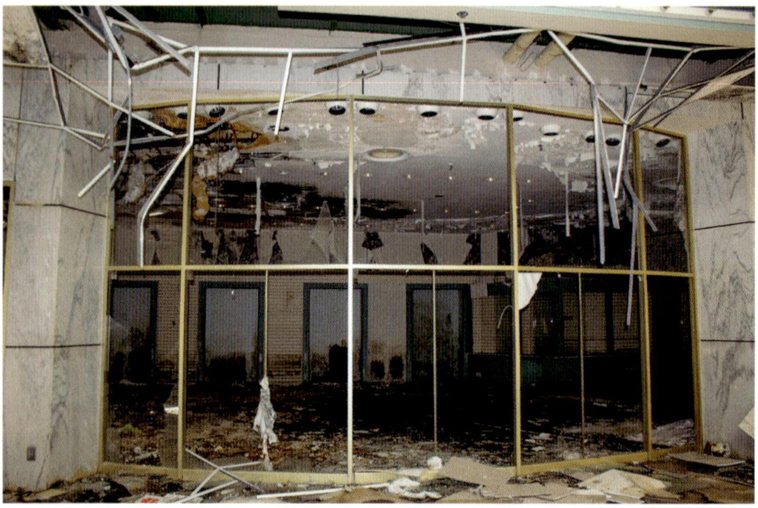

Ceiling collapsing in this shop.

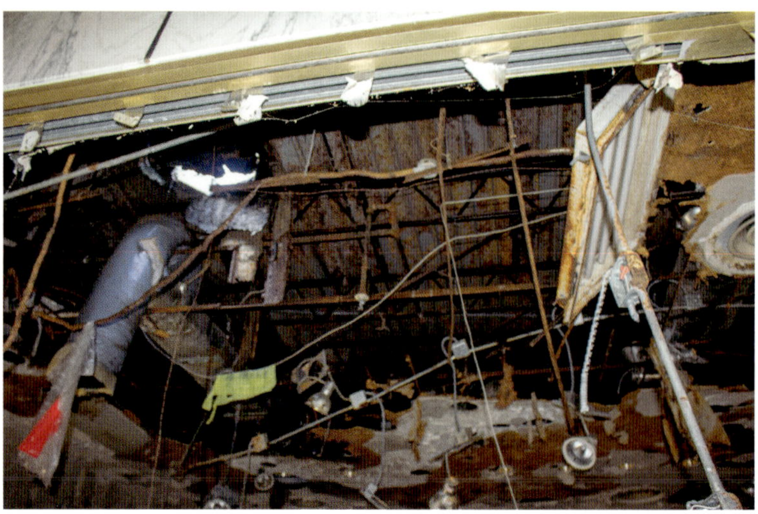

Ceiling collapsing shown.

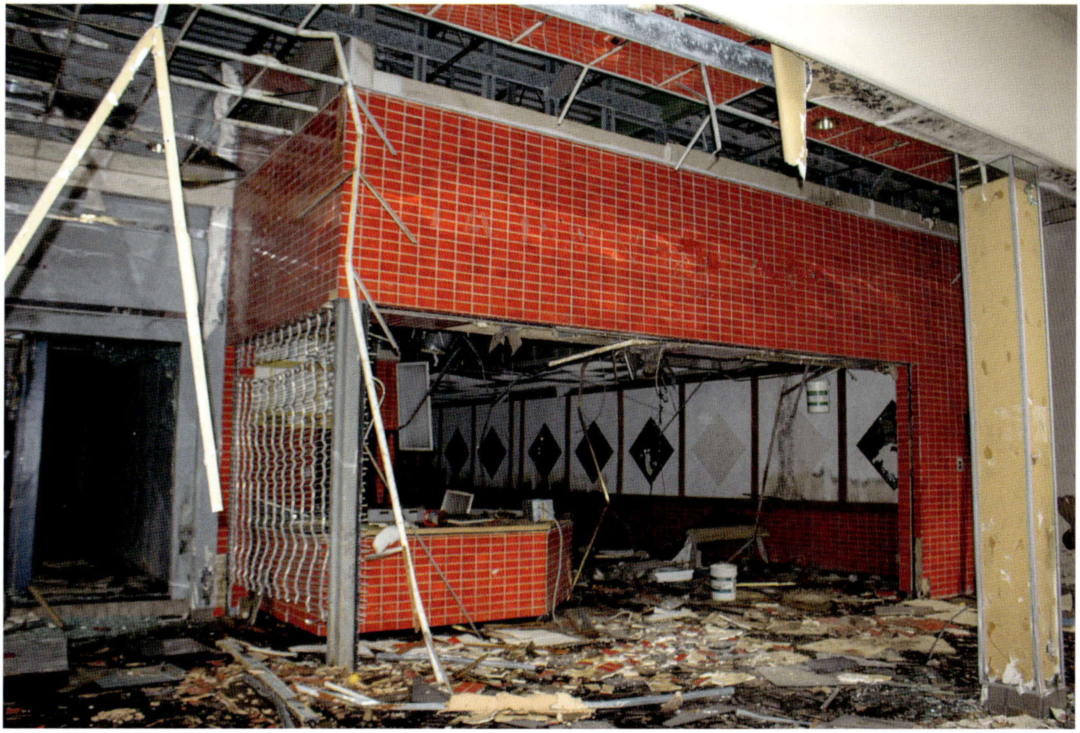

Parkway Pizza was located here, later becoming a Vietnamese restaurant.

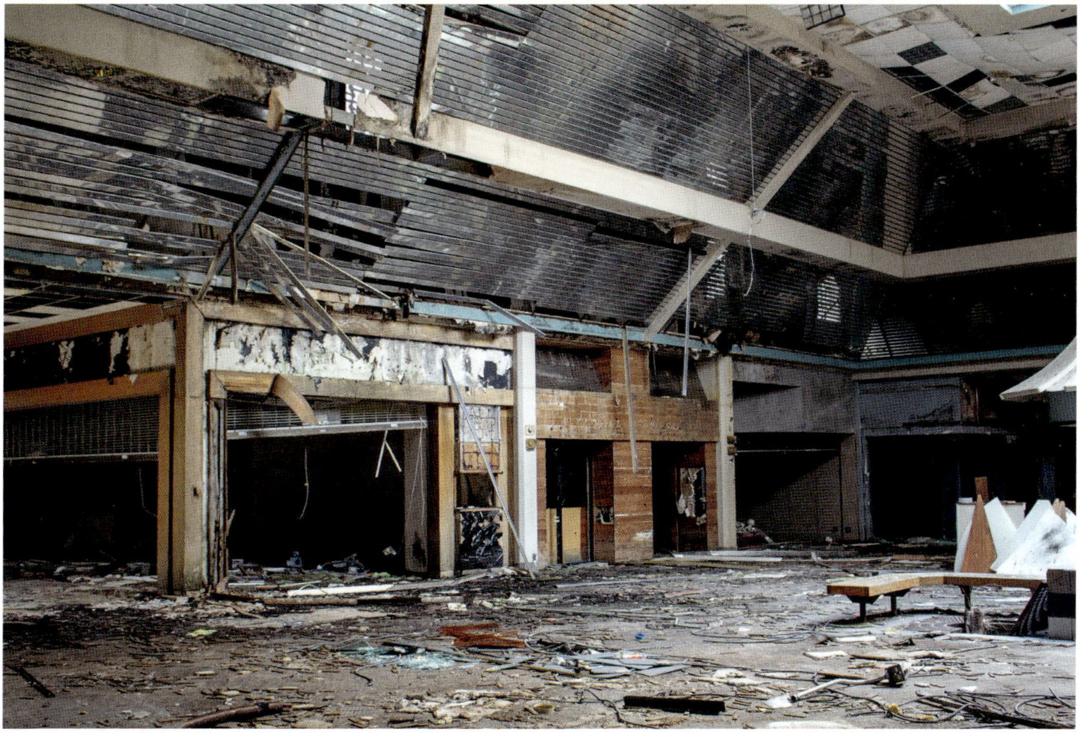

Former Calhoun's Jewelers on the far left.

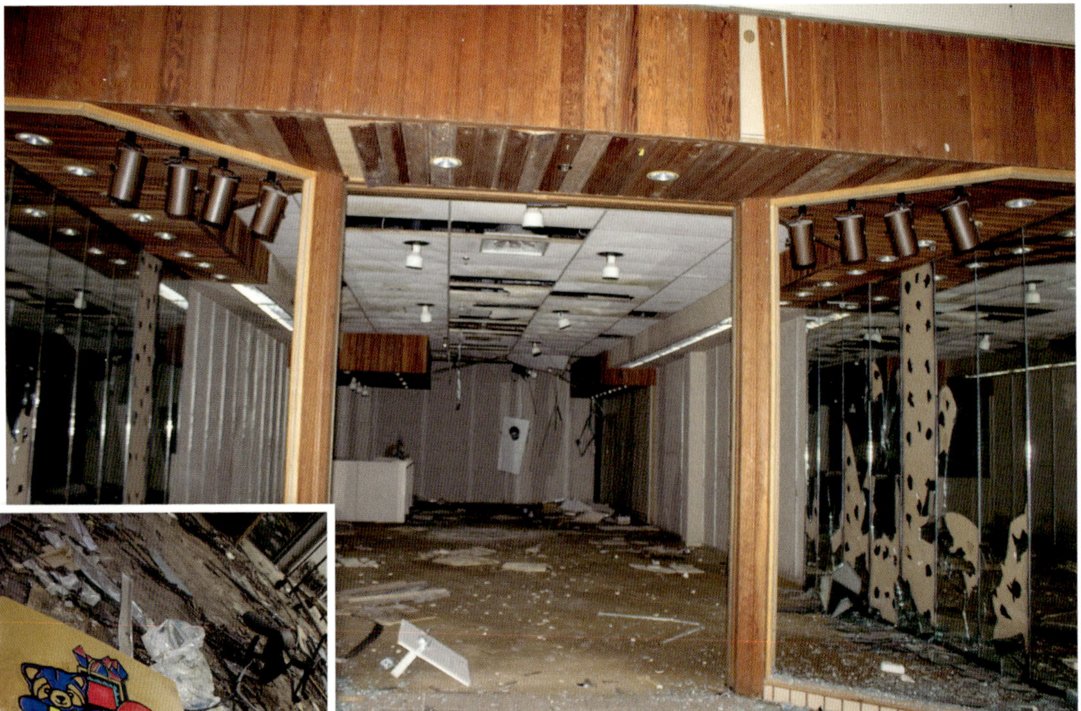

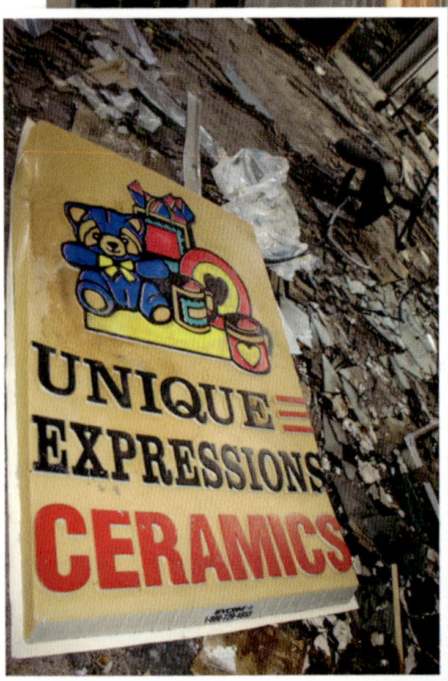

The mirrors have all been broken out of this shop.
Inset: Unique Expressions Ceramics.

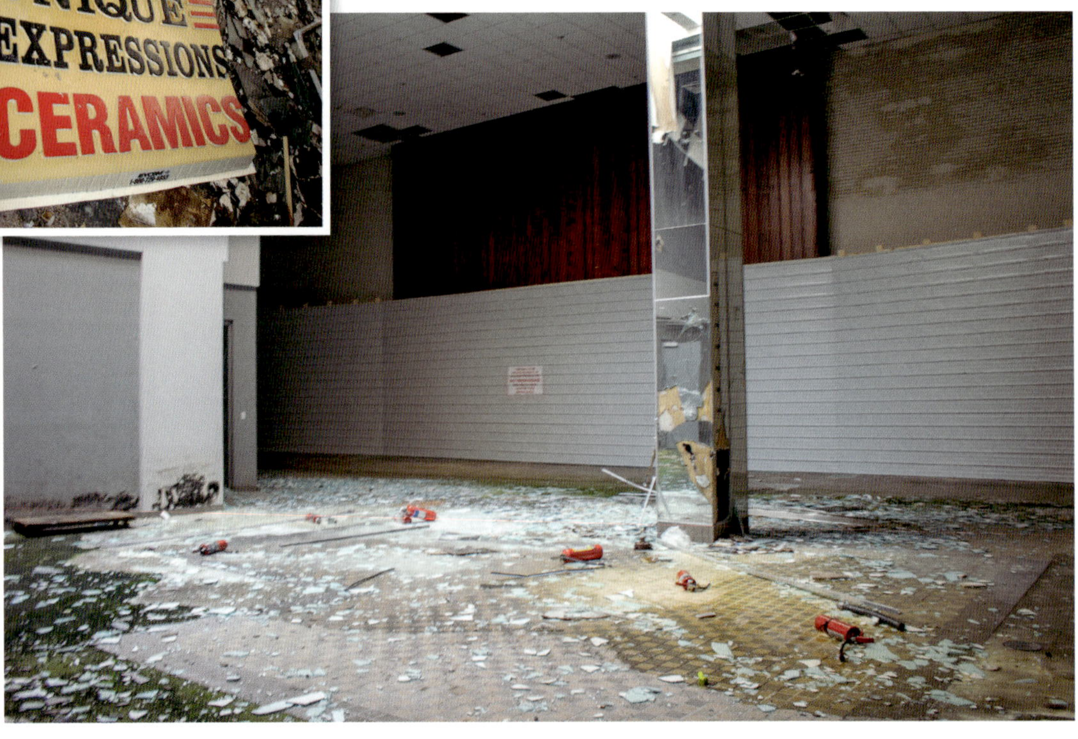

Glass and fire extinguishers scatter the floor in front of the dividing wall of Mainline Printing.

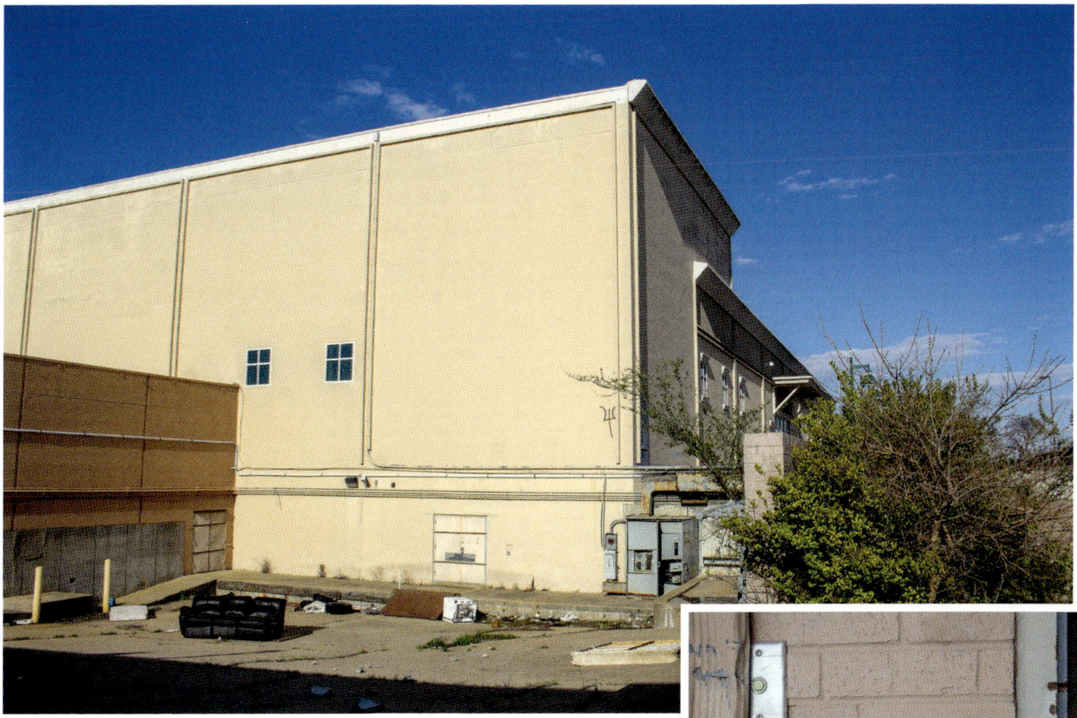

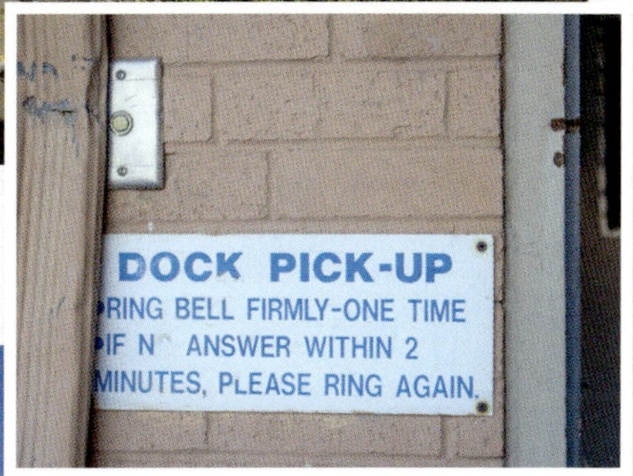
DOCK PICK-UP
RING BELL FIRMLY-ONE TIME
IF N ANSWER WITHIN 2
MINUTES, PLEASE RING AGAIN.

The back of the building has become a dumping ground.
Inset: Dock pick-up.

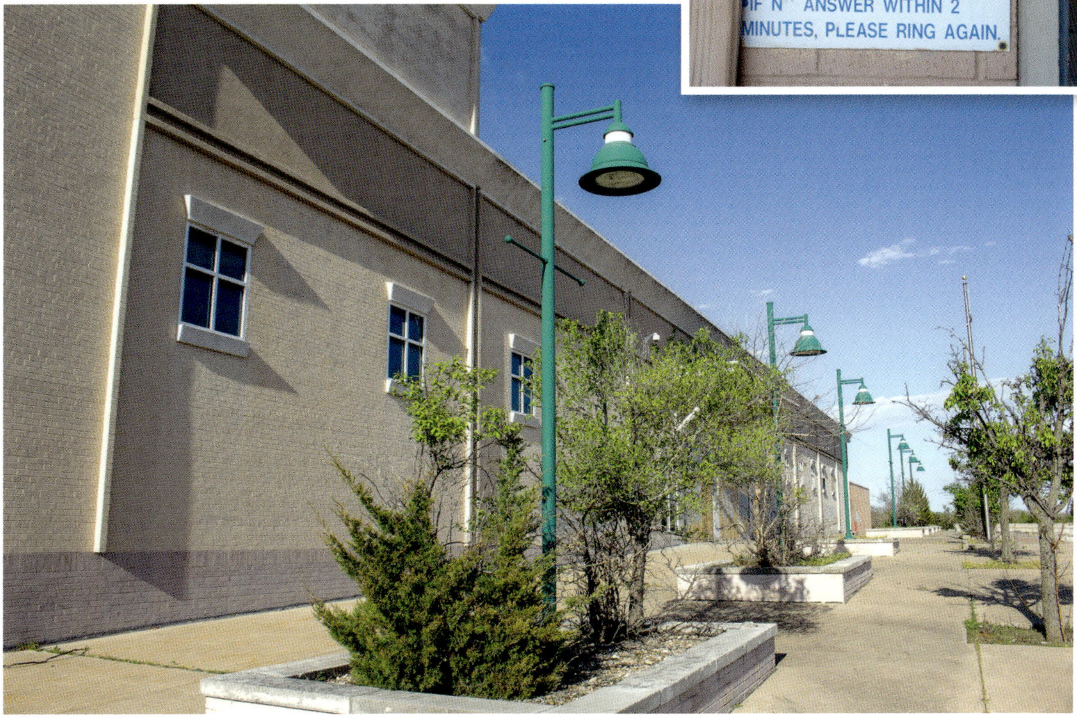

Lights strewn down the side entrance.

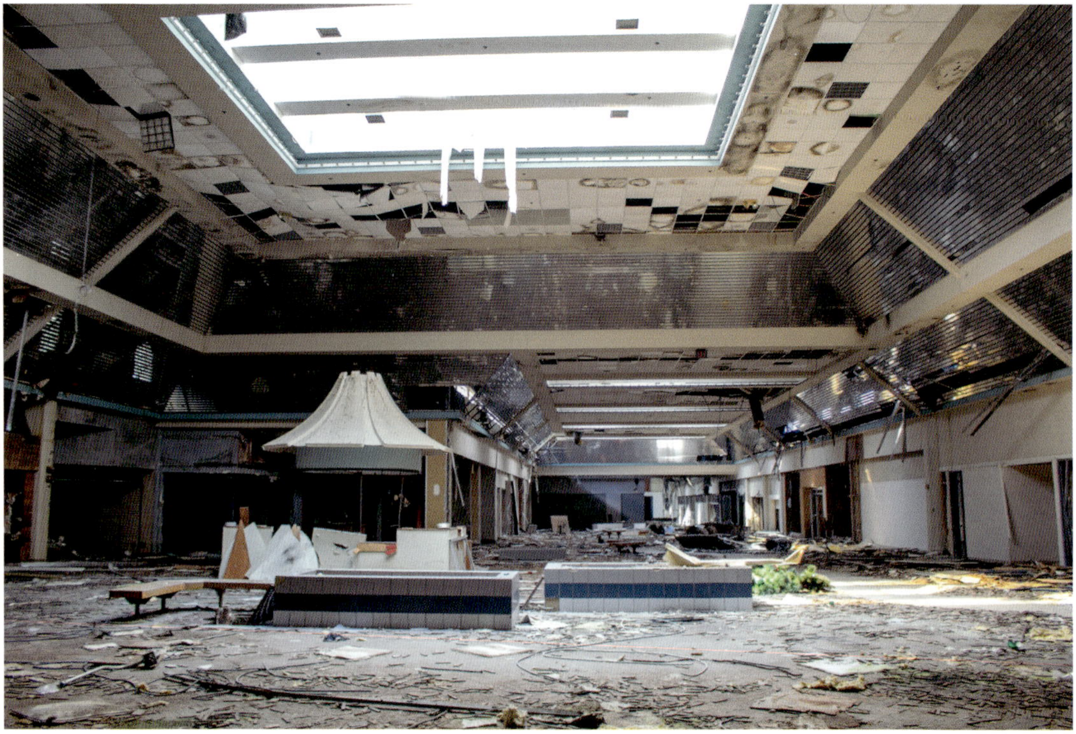

Where good things happened .

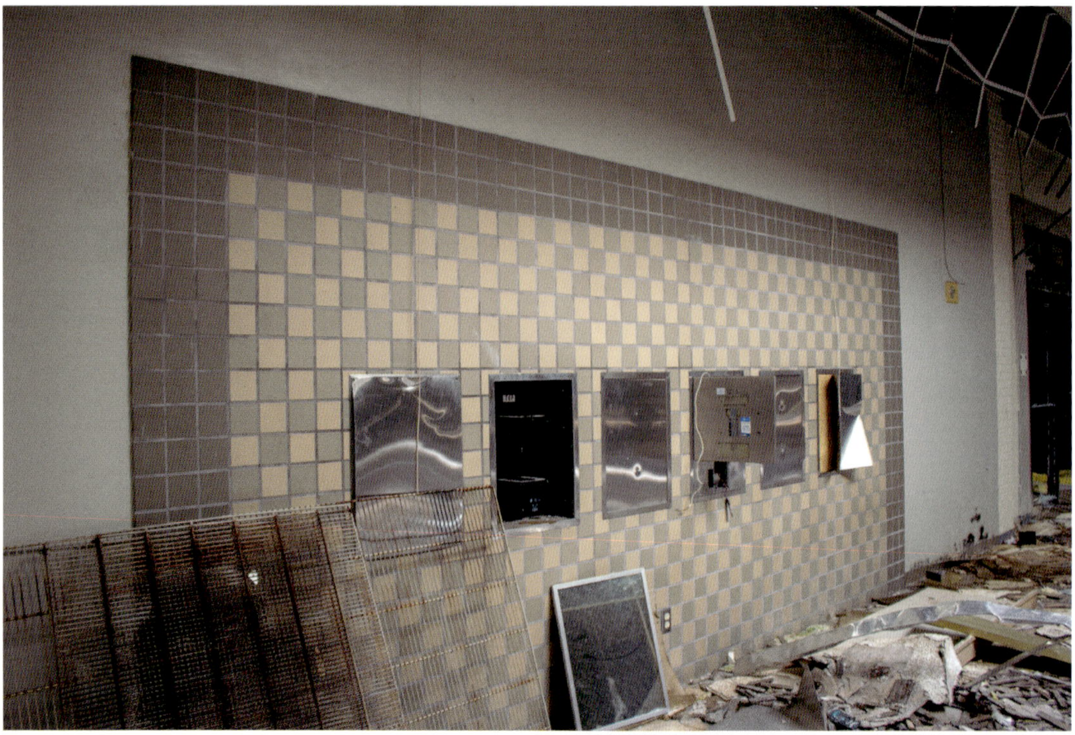

White Lakes Mall.

6

EAST TOPEKA JUNIOR HIGH

East Topeka Junior High (ETJH) is a modern movement/art deco school built in 1935-36. Walter Glover, who designed many other historic buildings in Topeka, designed the breathtaking structure which would cost a total of $380,000 after being completed. The two-story, U-shaped, remarkable school was constructed by architects Cuthbert & Suehrk and Bowers & Ingram, using poured concrete clad with varying shades of buff brick with areas of carved limestone. The facade is made up of a three-story tower with the words "East Topeka Junior High" carved above the doorway. The second story contains three windows with carved limestone above them and the rest of the tower is a vent leading from the windows to the peak of the tower. Office space and the former library are located on the front of the building's first story. The rear wings are filled with classrooms that possess beautiful fir floors, while the hallways throughout the structure have classic terrazzo flooring. The junior high served grades seven through nine and was made up of mostly minority students.

Shout it loud East Topeka
Shout it loud shout it strong
The Bulldog growls to the sky
Go get that ball and bring it back
For the orange and the black
East Topeka my own Jr high

That was one of the encouraging chants students and cheerleaders shouted courtside as the Bulldogs played many of their basketball games. In the early years, school colors were brown and gold, while the last twenty years of the Bulldogs, colors were orange and black. Throughout the 1940s, Topeka High's Black basketball team,

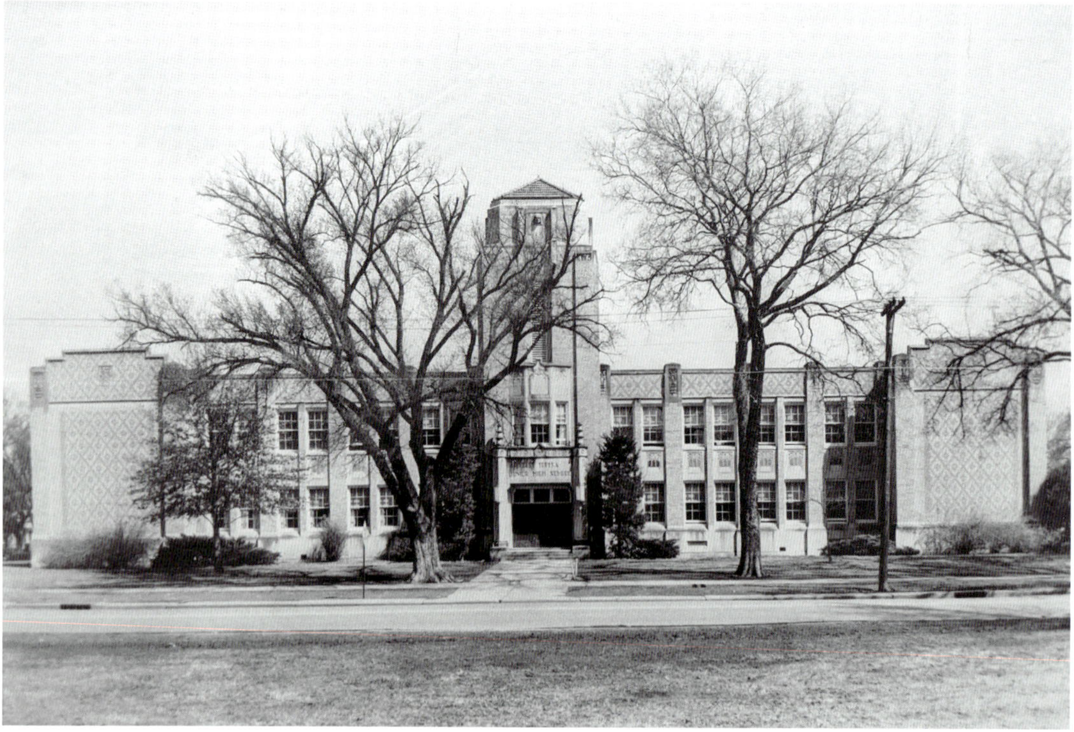

Picture that hung in the main hallway. Presented to ETJH by E-Teen Club in 1965. [*Brice Smith*]

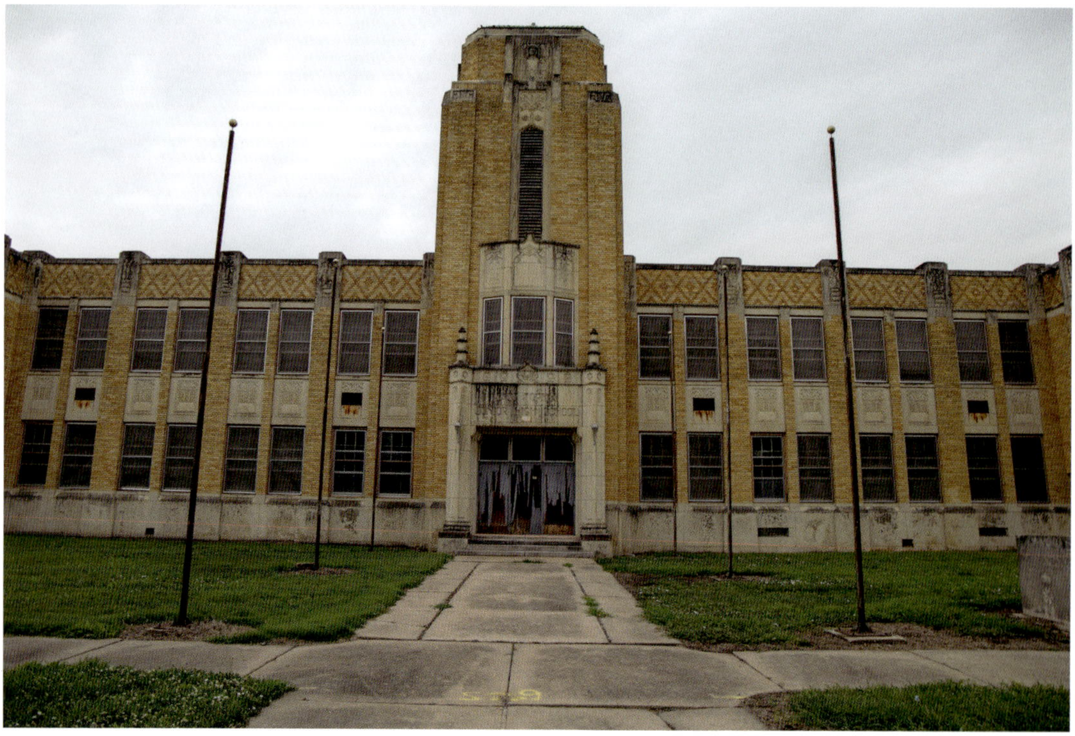

The large trees that once stood on each side of the entrance are now gone.

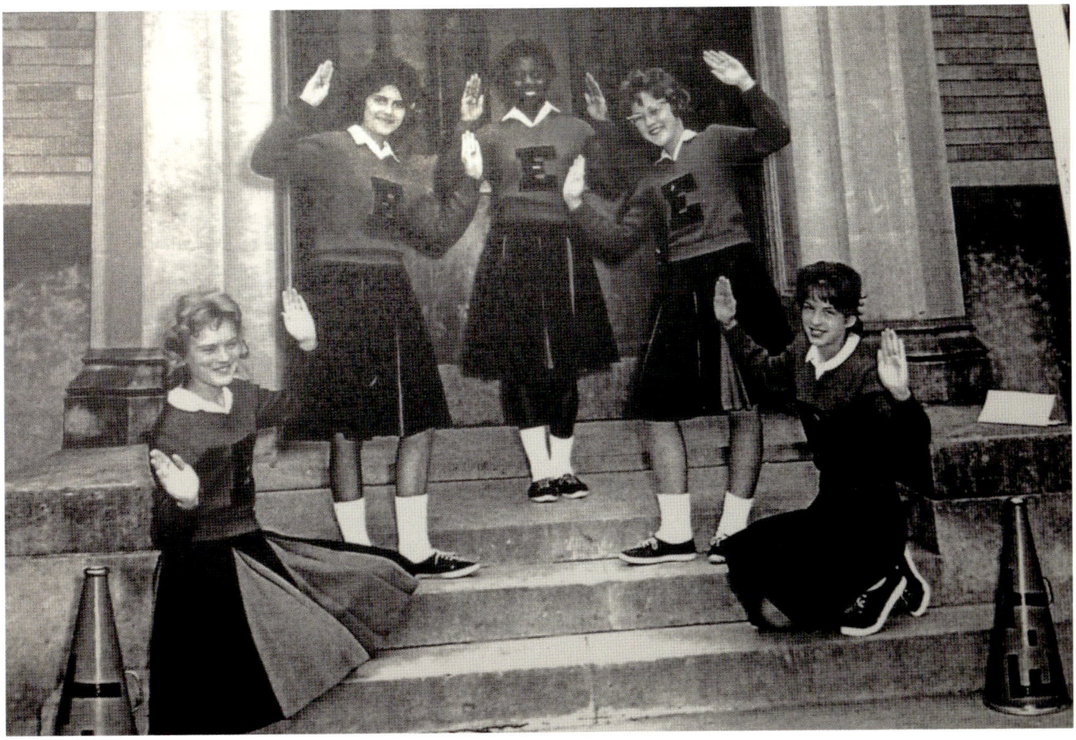

East Topeka Junior High Cheerleaders 1963. [*Vernon McFalls*]

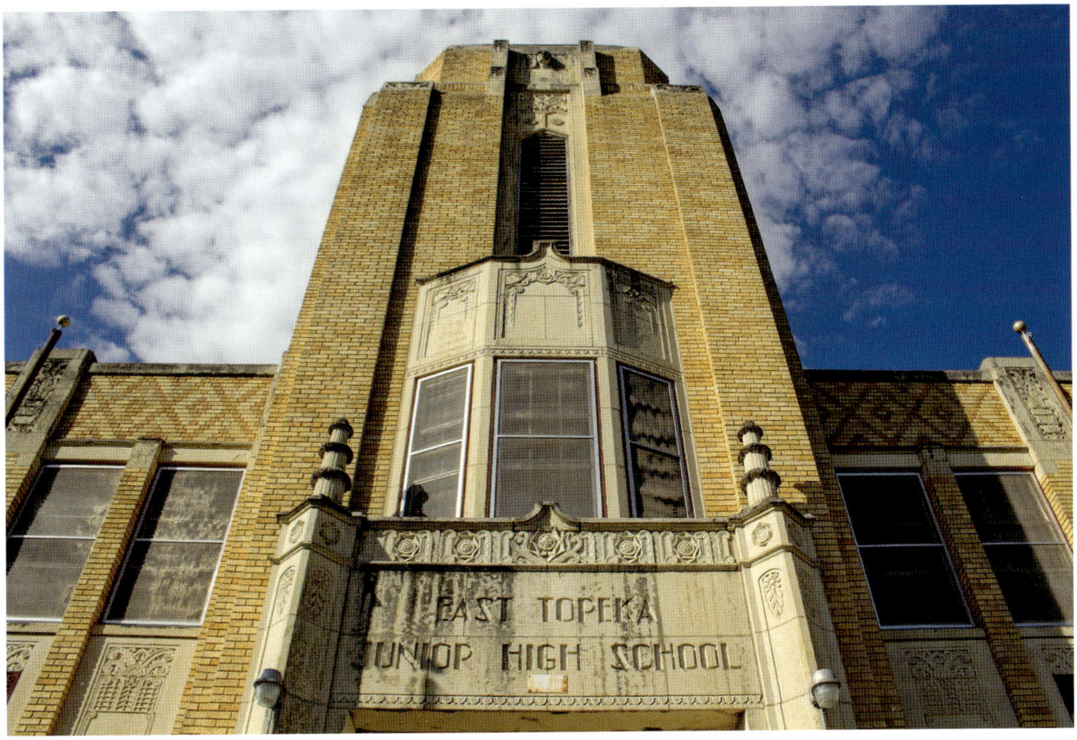

Modern movement/art deco features with East Topeka Junior High carved into limestone.

known as the Ramblers, had home games and practices in the East Topeka Junior High gym. The Ramblers and the Bulldogs were known as some of the most skilled basketball players in Topeka. It wasn't just basketball that they were good at; the Bulldogs had highlights in track and baseball as well.

Staff at ETJH were caring, creative, and genuinely wanted students to succeed. "People don't realize how amazing some of these teachers were. I hesitate to say they were all saints, but by God, they believed in what they did. I miss that a lot these days," said Vernon McFalls, who attended from '67 to '70. Mr. Otto Bodenhausen, known by some as Bud, had an extensive academic teaching background, being principal at Sumner Elementary earlier in his career and later at East Topeka Junior High. He loved teaching and finding new and innovative ways to improve the education system. He shortened class periods to allow students to add an elective and created a Boys Food course, which quickly gained popularity. "He was a fun person. Bud was known as a sort of a matchmaker and would set new teachers up with meet and greets when the school year started. He was responsible for a number of weddings among his young teachers," said Elizabeth Svercl.

Malcolm Smith was a vice principal, coach, and math teacher in his twenty-six-year career at ETJH from 1954 to 1980, when the school closed. "Malcolm Smith was a great man first, a great math teacher, and a great basketball coach. The best coach in the city at the time in my opinion. Soft-spoken, he worked us hard!" said former student Vernon Mcfalls. After talking with his children and former students I could tell how much he cared about his job and how much he cared about his students.

> I have great memories of East Topeka Junior High School during my dad's teaching years. Although I never attended the school, I spent a lot of time there because my dad, Malcolm Smith, was a math teacher there. He coached different sports at East Topeka including basketball and track. On weekends he would take my brothers and I with him and we would play basketball in the gym while he worked. My brothers and I were also given jobs moving books from classrooms to the auditorium after school ended and then from the auditorium back to the classrooms before school started.
>
> Brice Smith, son of Mr. Smith

> I vividly remember being in the gym to watch weekly inter-city basketball games since Dad was the Basketball Coach. I can still smell the popcorn from the concession stand and I remember feeling hot in there even though it was winter outside. In Junior High I remember going with Dad on the weekends when he went in to get caught up on grading papers. He would set up the trampoline for me and my brothers to jump on by the gym in the hall.

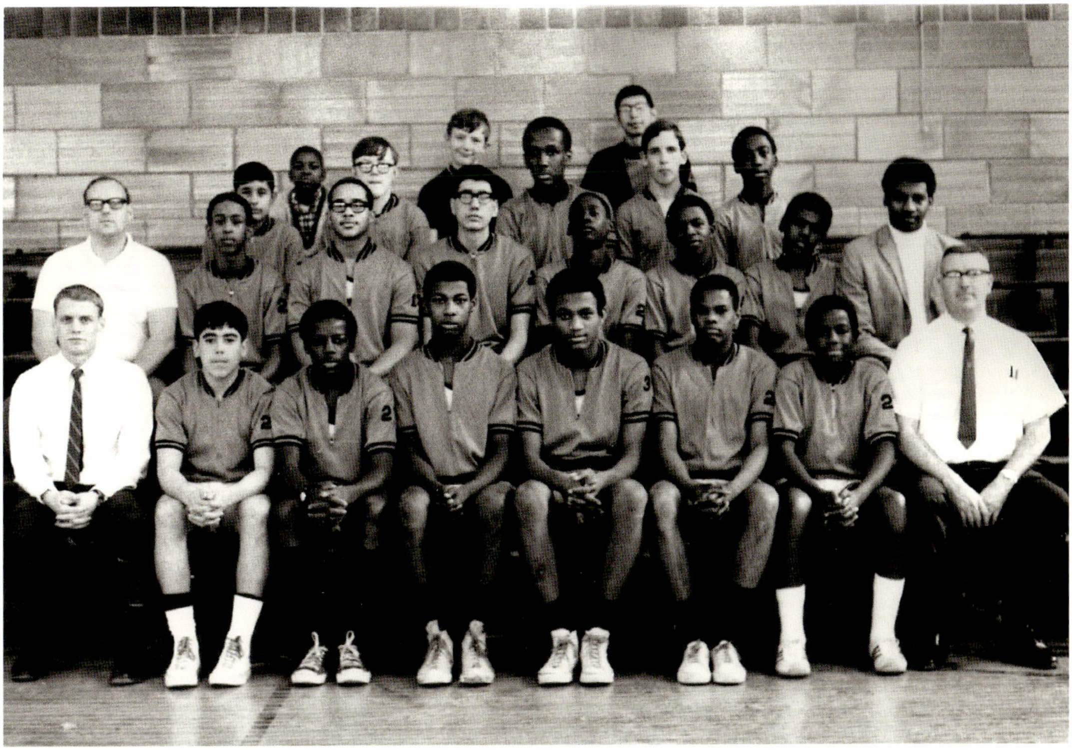

ETJH Basketball Team 1968-69. Coach Malcolm Smith pictured right. [*Courtesy of Brice Smith*]

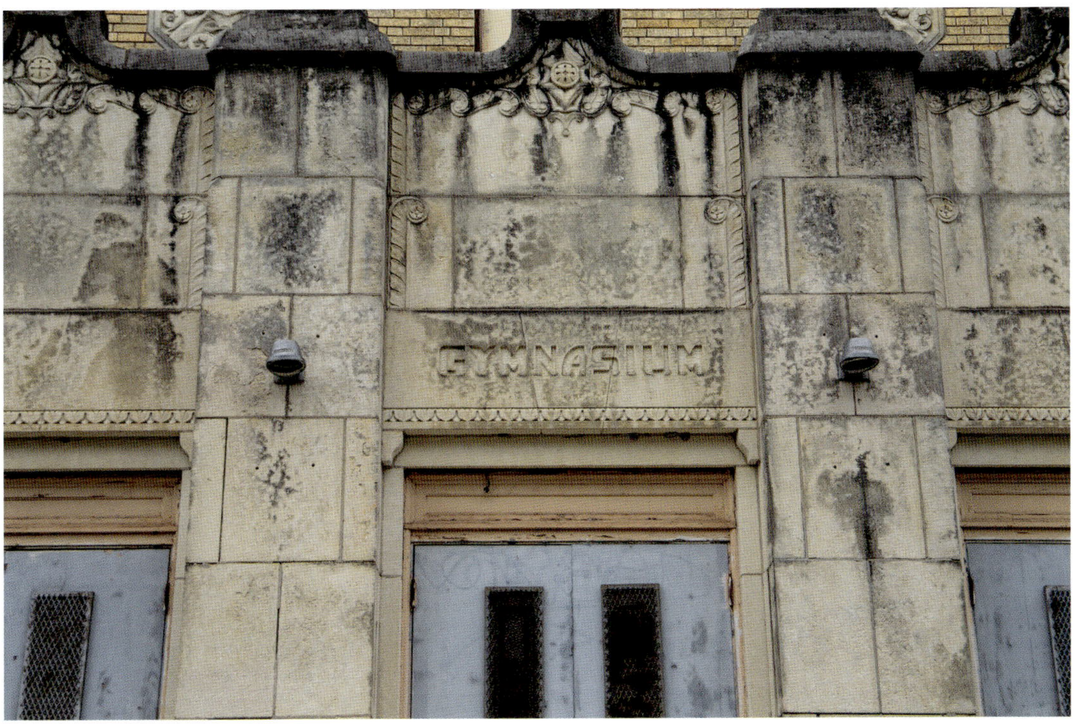

Gymnasium engraving.

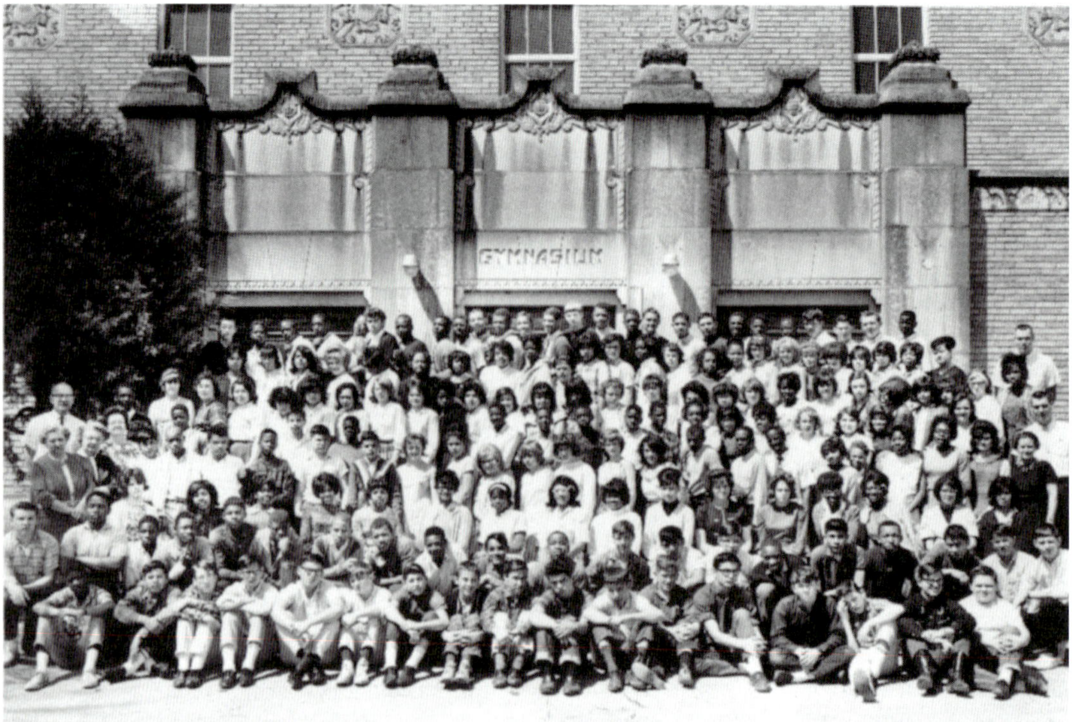

Class of 1965. [*Vernon McFalls*]

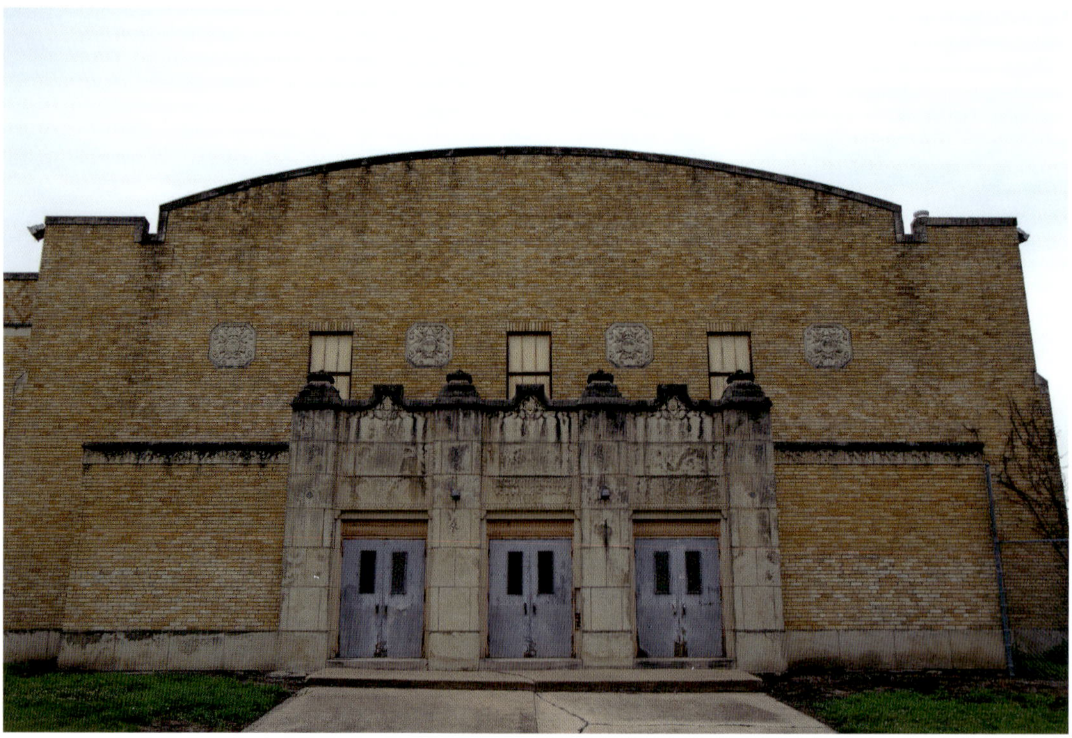

Gymnasium doors where class photos were taken.

> He loved teaching at East Topeka, he always talked about a supportive parent base and good kids. I remember when he decided to dye shoelaces bright orange for the basketball team. Other schools had parent groups that had more money and those types of things were purchased for their teams. Dad had my mom and a Maytag washer and dryer to do the work. When there wasn't enough money to hire buses for away games, my parents bought a used VW bus, Dad got a chauffeur's license so he could drive the team to away activities. He hated the sort of class system that existed in the school system but was determined that it would not impact his kids if he could possibly change things. Cliff Alfrey, another East Topeka staff person, used to make the most wonderfully decorated cakes for everyone's birthday. For my dad, the cake was appropriately named "Big Mac" and it looked just like one!
>
> Elizabeth Svercl, daughter of Malcolm Smith

The community within East Topeka Junior High and surrounding neighborhoods were welcoming and embraced each other. In 1970, East Topeka United Methodist Church sponsored a teenage drop-in center every school day from 3:30 p.m. to 5 p.m., because they had noticed students standing around looking bored after classes. "We are very tight, we're all still friends to this day. I think the school's infrastructure helped all of us accept one another in our diversity. The three years I went there were some of my best memories," said Melody Oxy, a former cheerleader at ETJH. Former classmates continue to embrace each other forty years after the school's closing, holding yearly reunions and some still talking on a regular basis.

Even though the *Brown v. Board of Education* verdict was announced twenty-six years earlier, racial bias was still active in Topeka schools. Busing for integration had not been used and allowed for students to attend schools of their choice, causing an imbalance in minority and white students. East Topeka Junior High had a minority enrollment of 71%, and most white students had transferred to other schools while minority students often times did not have the transportation to move schools. The school district put in place a long-range plan designed to partially solve the racial imbalance particularly at the junior high level. ETJH was one of five junior highs closing. Starting in the 1980-81 school year, students would go to one of the four remaining junior highs and two additional ones.

The school was privately sold to a couple for $50,000 in 1987; unfortunately, it was discovered that it had asbestos and due to the hazmat conditions for removal it would cost too much for them to remove the asbestos and make repairs to the school. It was reimagined in an East Topeka Neighborhood Revitalization Plan in April of 2002 as a housing complex for seniors. An article dated September 21, 2005, addresses that gang activity in the area made it unsafe for the planned senior housing complex that would reside in the East Topeka Junior High. A subcommittee therefore rejected a proposal for the city to condemn the school and turn it over to a local developer, Pioneer Group Inc. "They're going to be right in the line of fire," councilwoman Sylvia Ortiz said. It is currently said to be owned by a church and undergoing renovations, but it is still unoccupied as of December 2020.

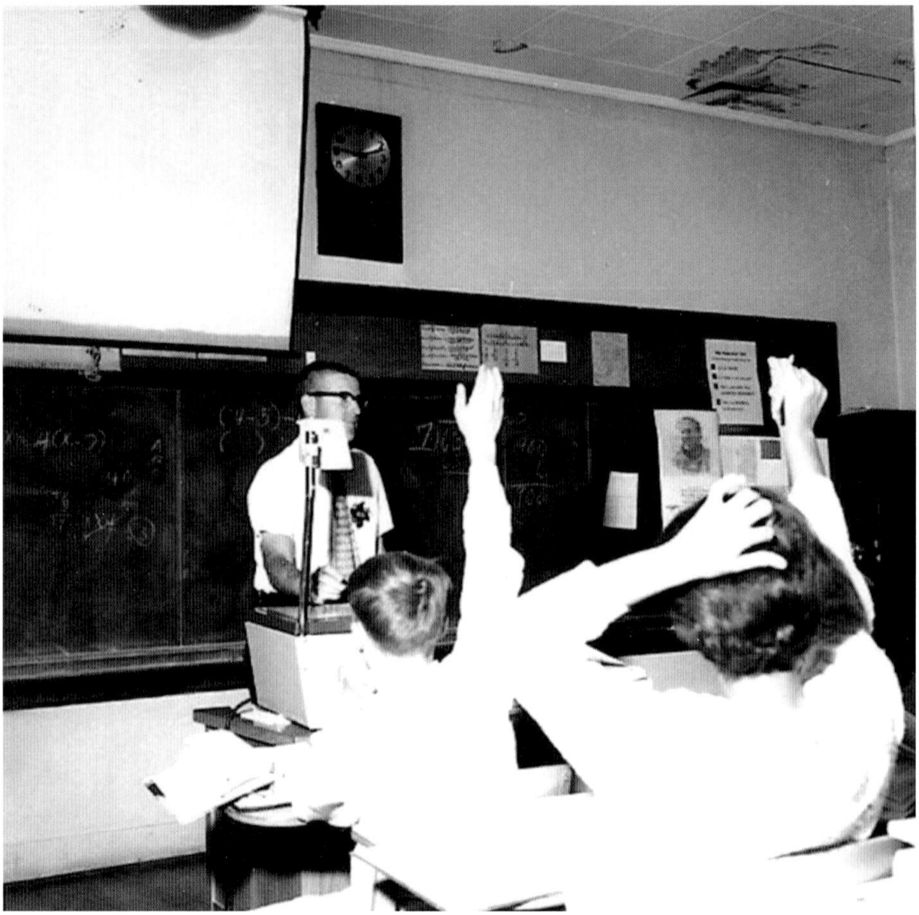

Malcolm Smith teaching in Room 204. [*Brice Smith*]

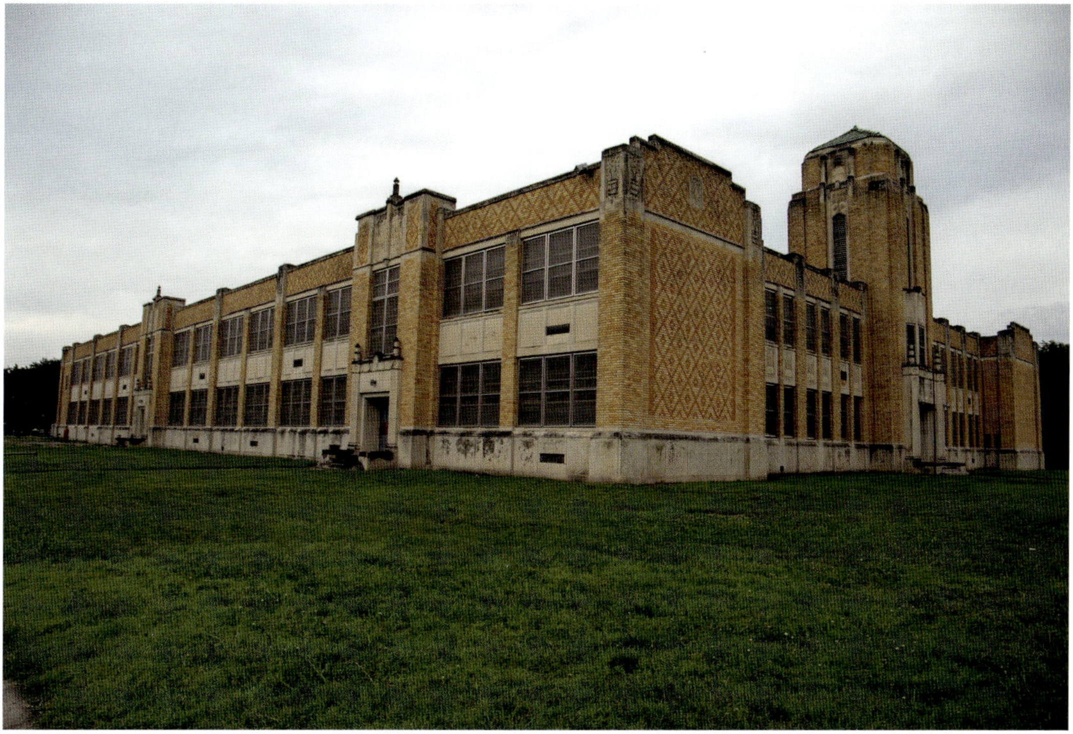

West side of ETJH.

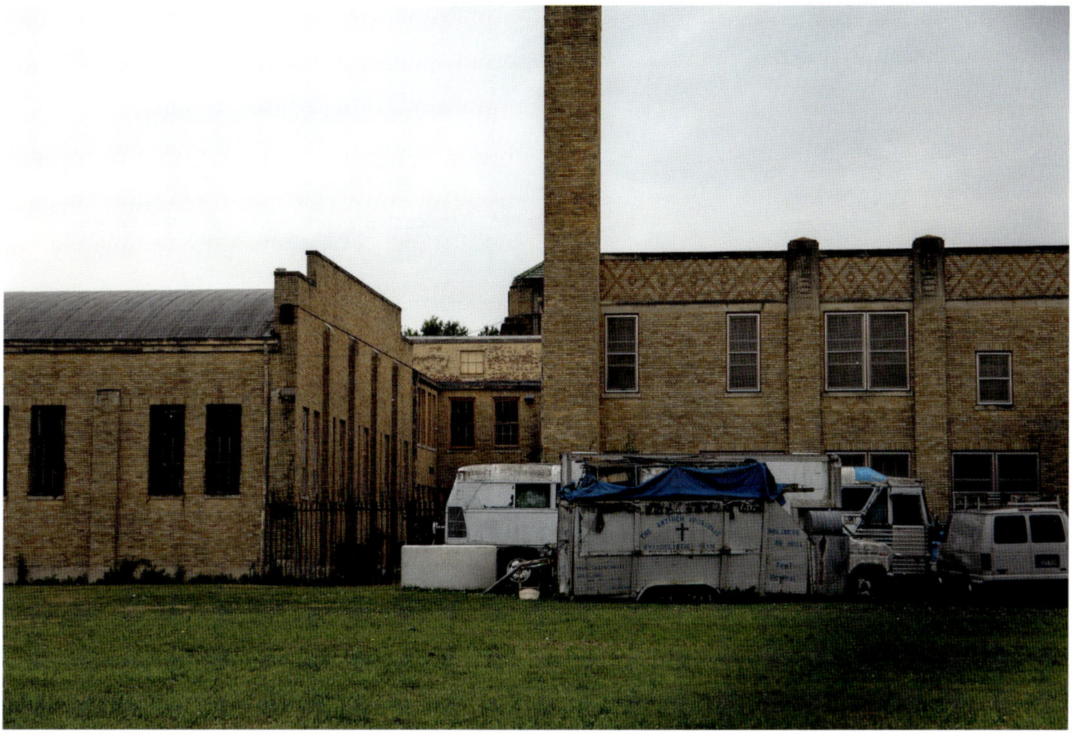

Church buses stored at the backside of the building.

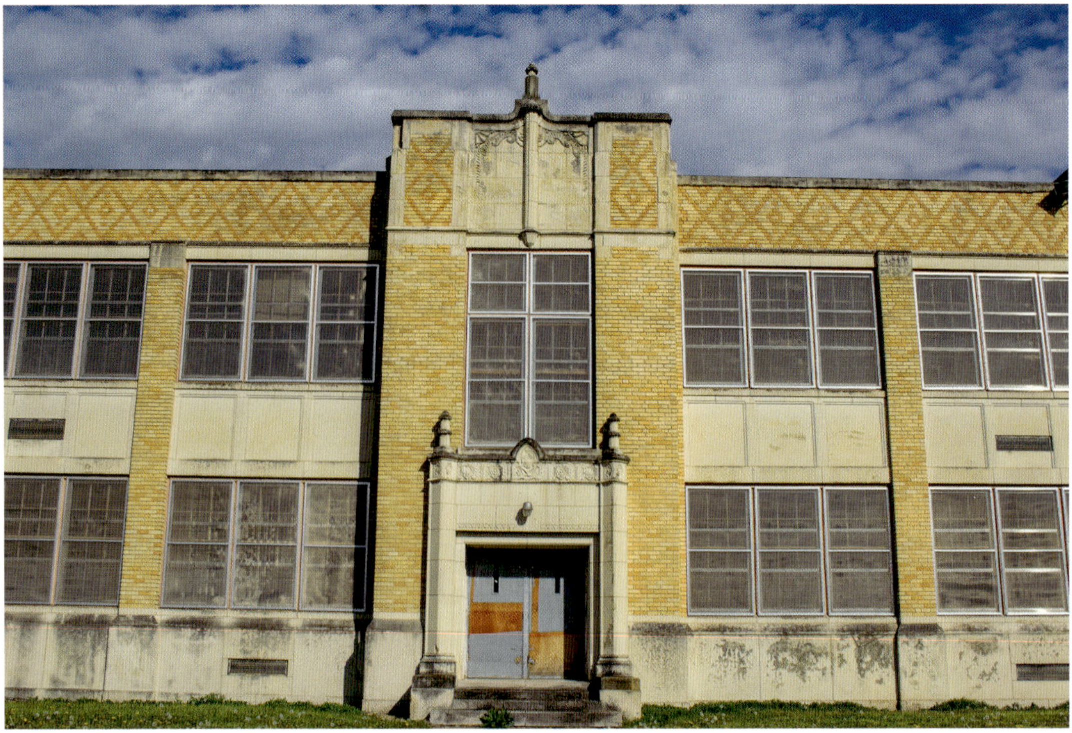

Entrance on the West side of building.

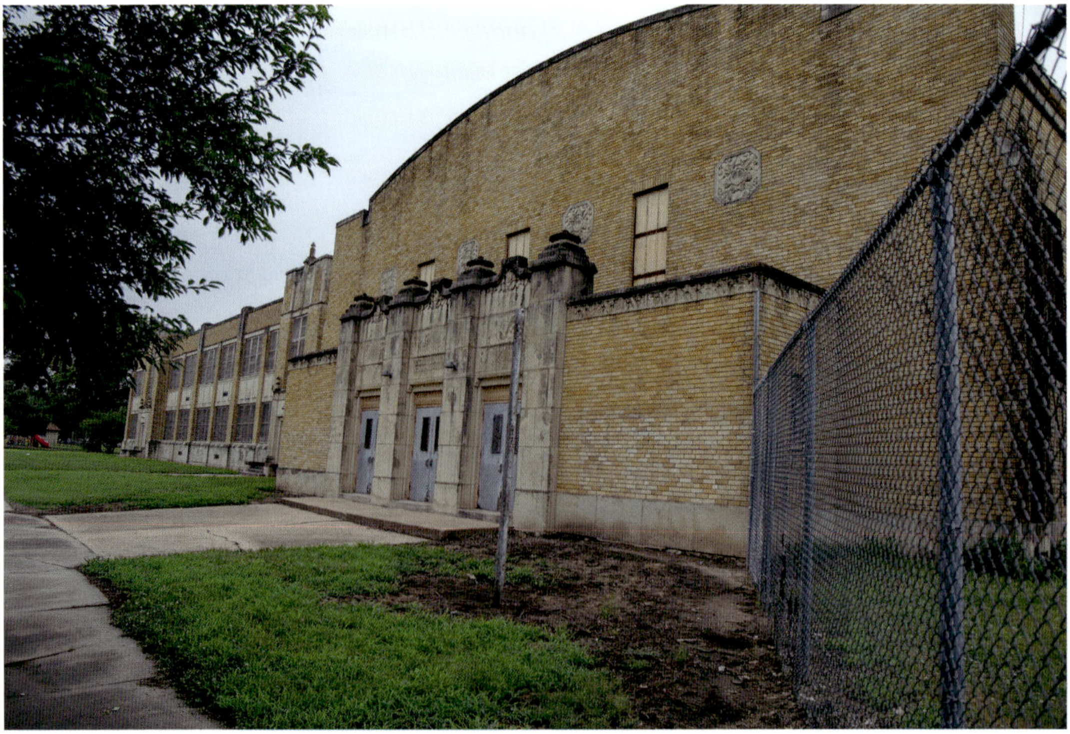

Gymnasium with playground to the right.

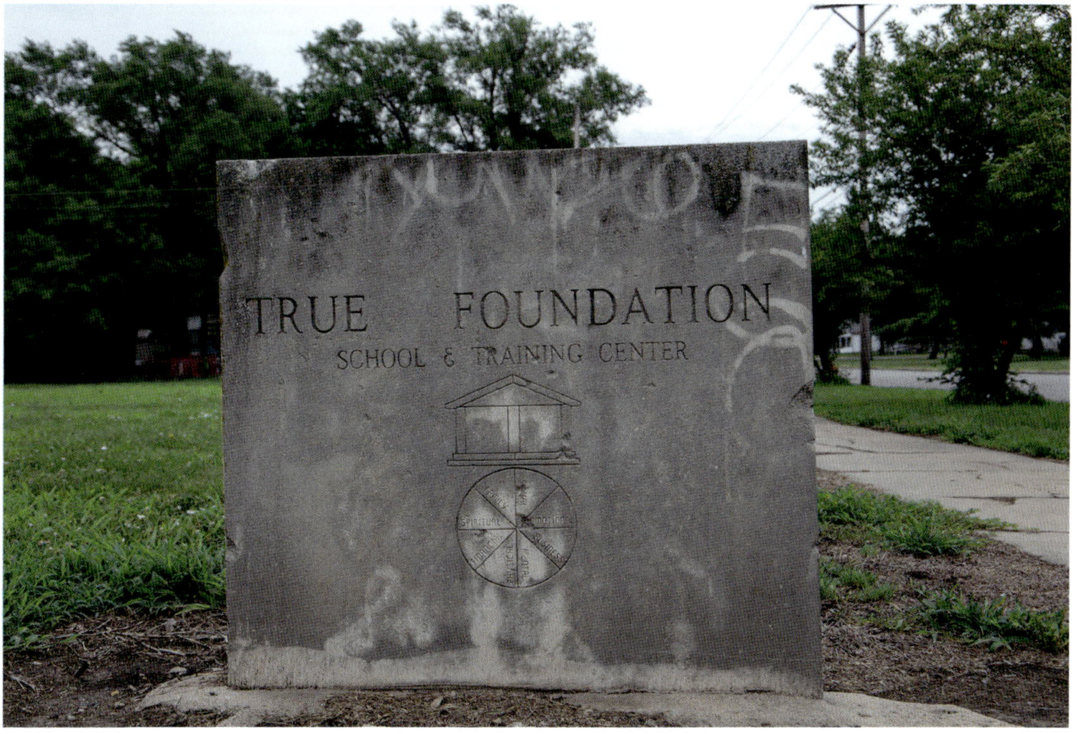

"True Foundation School & Training Center."

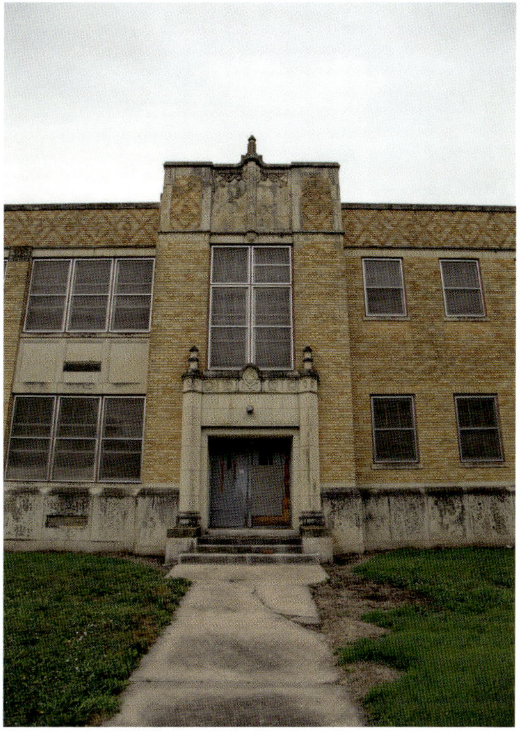

West entrance.

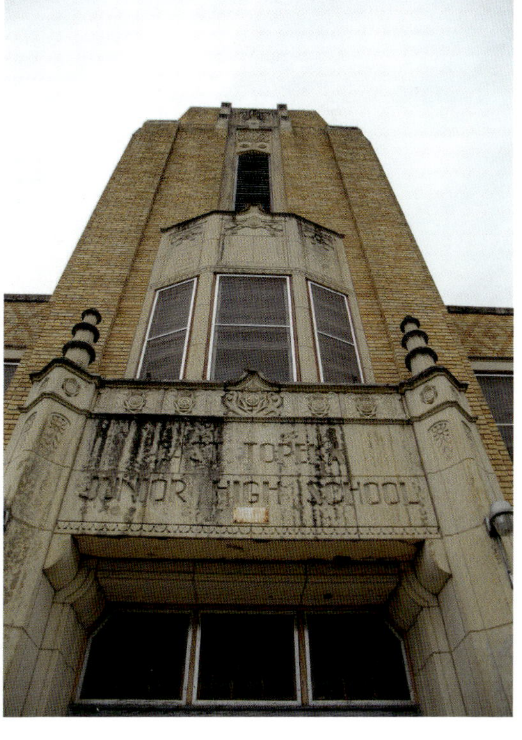

Main entrance.

7

HONORABLE MENTION TOPEKA STATE HOSPITAL

While this is a location very important to Topeka's history, especially in the world of mental health, I have plans to include it in my next book. For now, enjoy a few pictures of what is left of the campus and keep an eye out for my next publication!

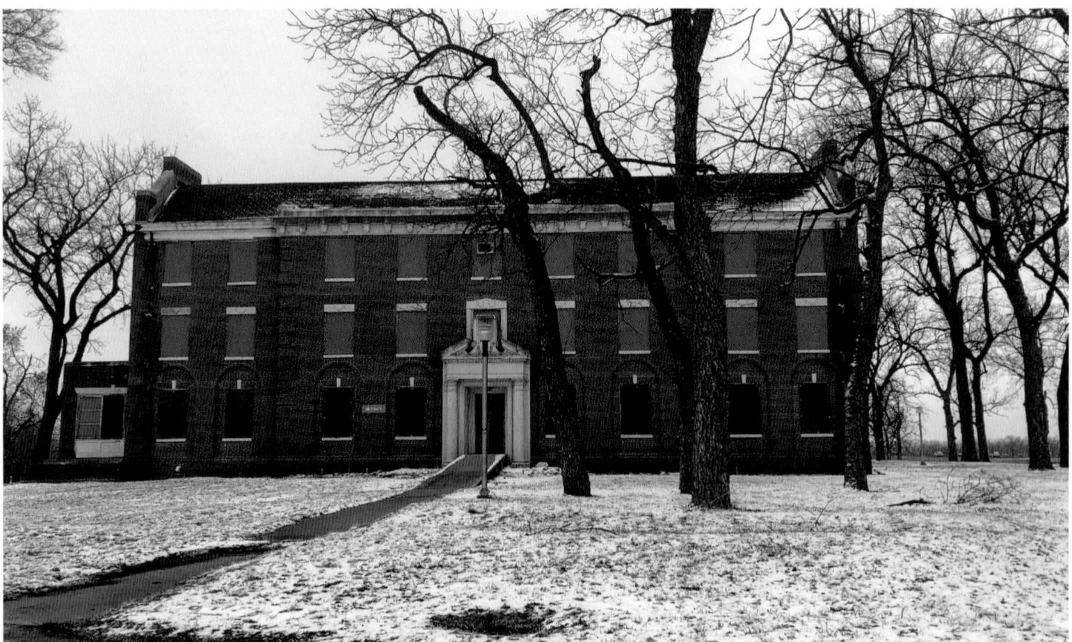

One of the last buildings left on the grounds.

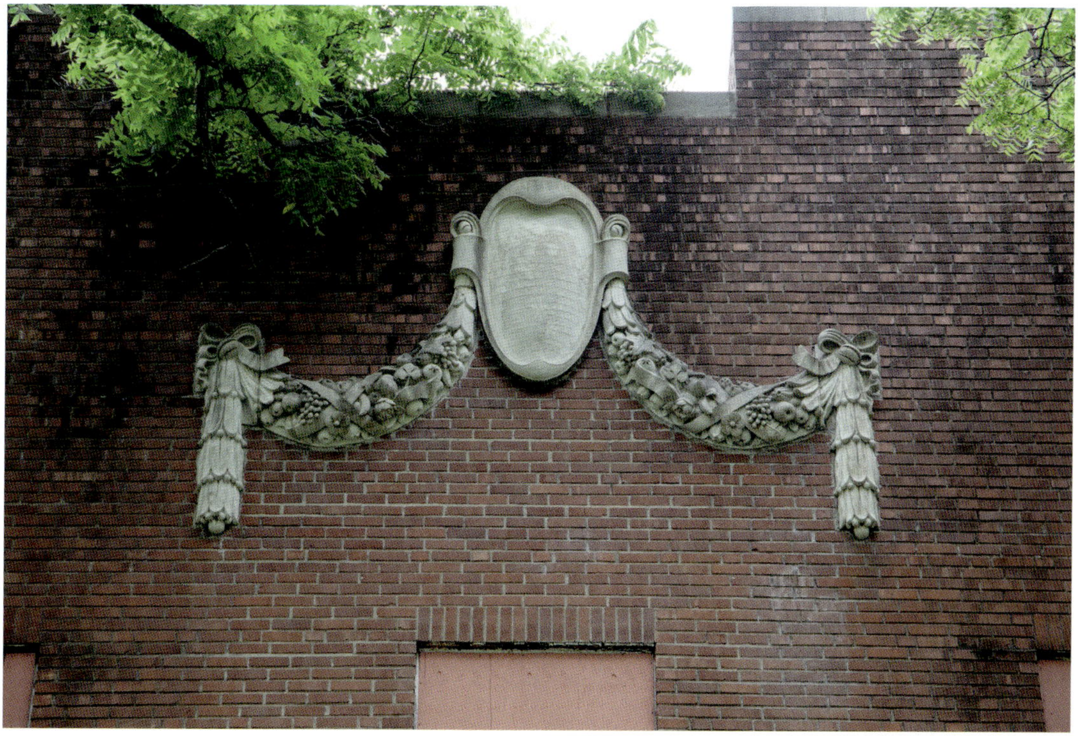

Intricate details line the top of the building.

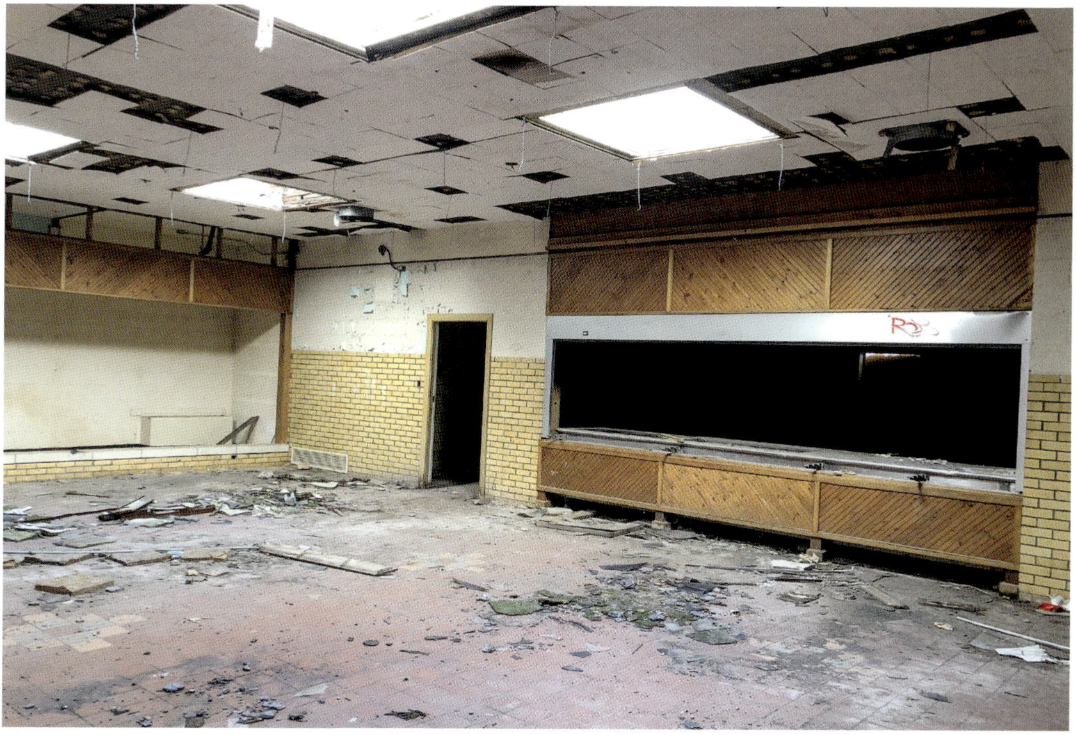

Cafeteria.

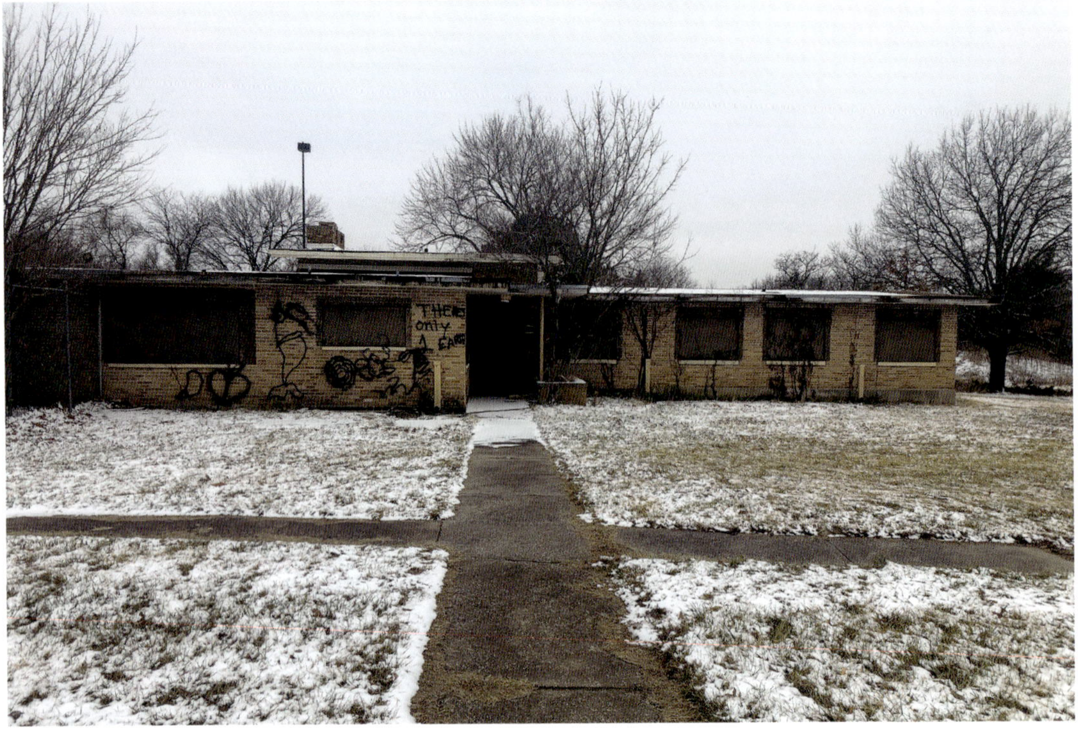

Snow and graffiti cover this building.

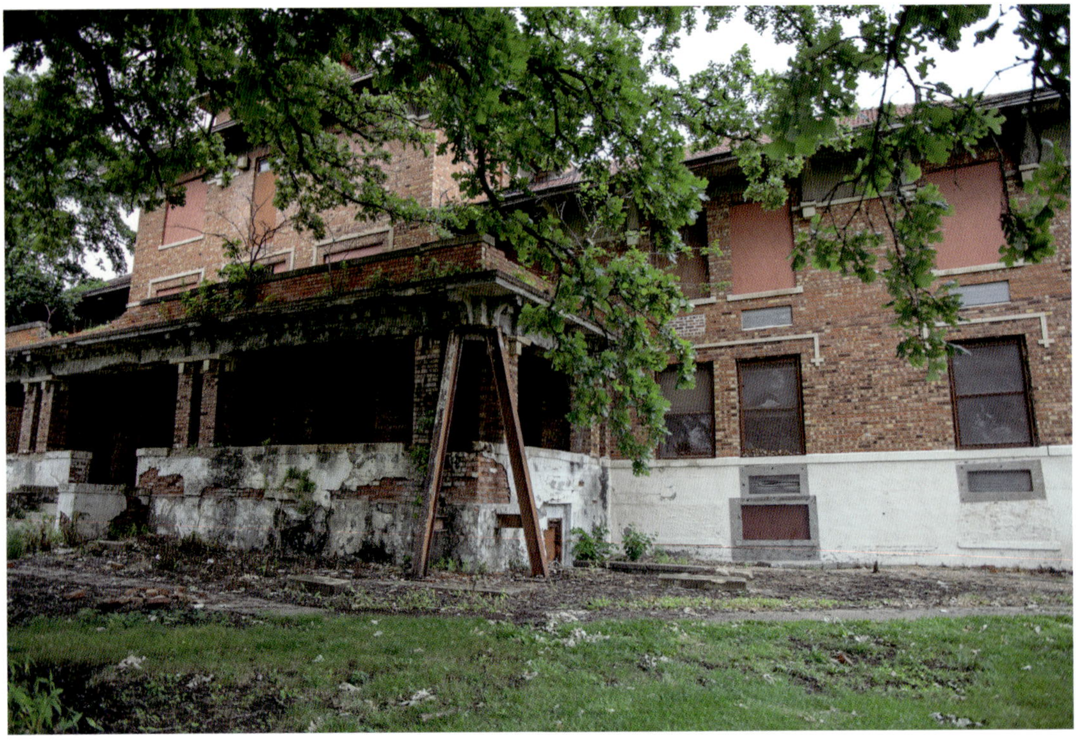

Steel braces this crumbling building.

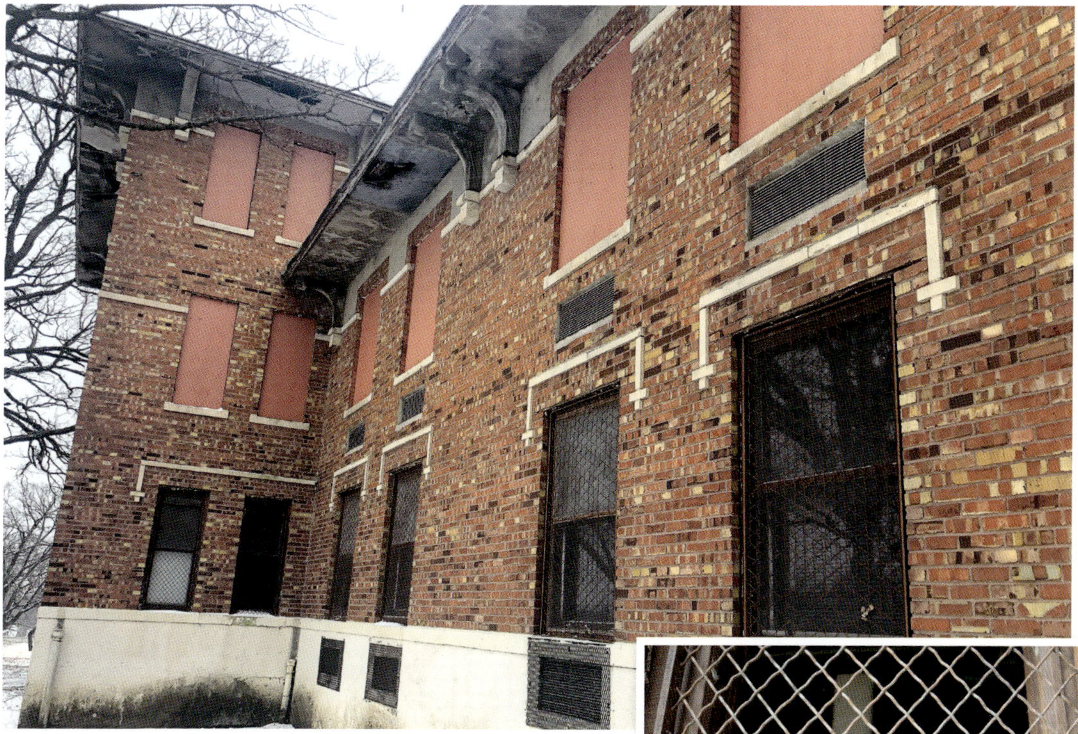

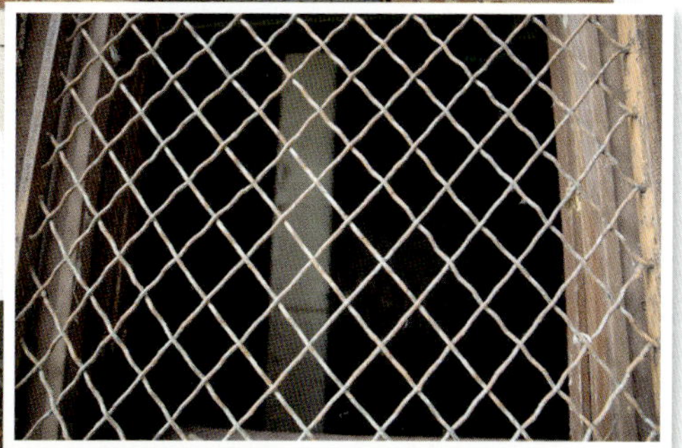

The roof is starting to rot. *Inset:* In an attempt to keep transients and amateur artists out, this window is covered with wire.

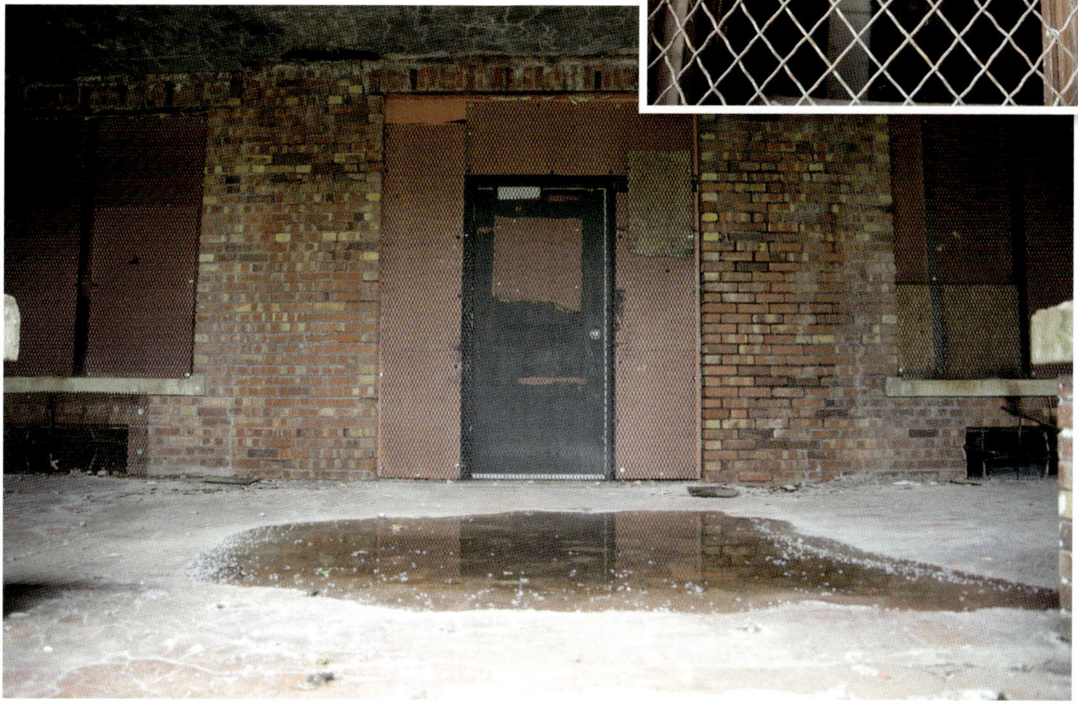

Locked up.

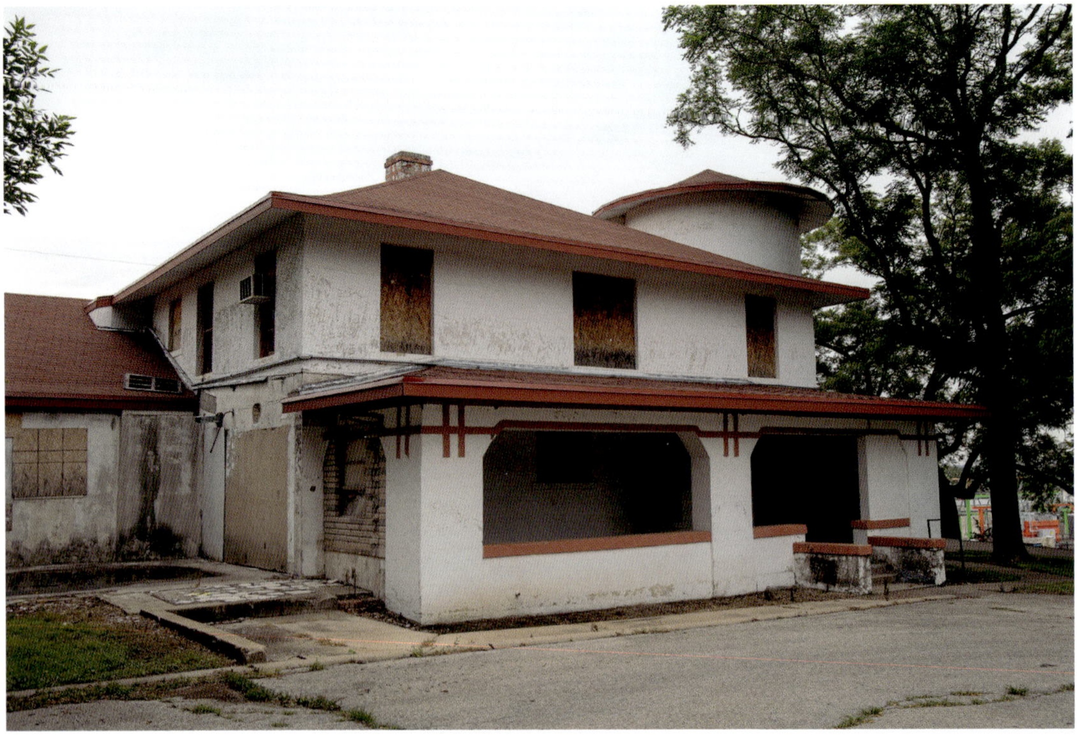

Dairy barn.

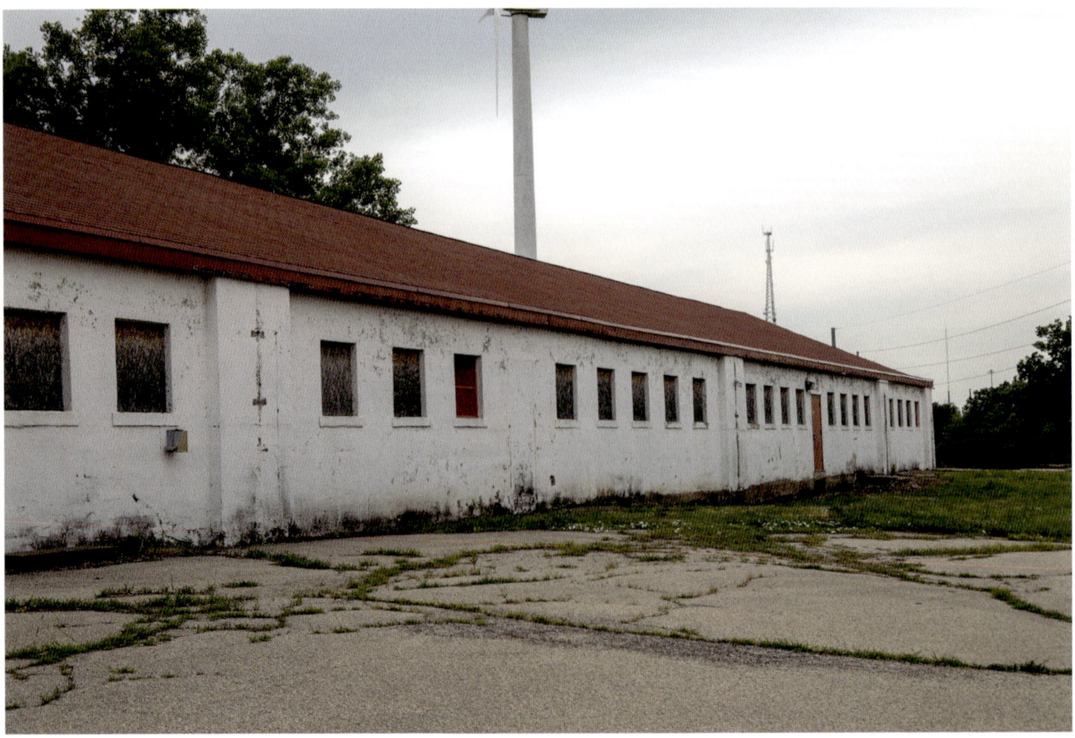

The barn had many windows.

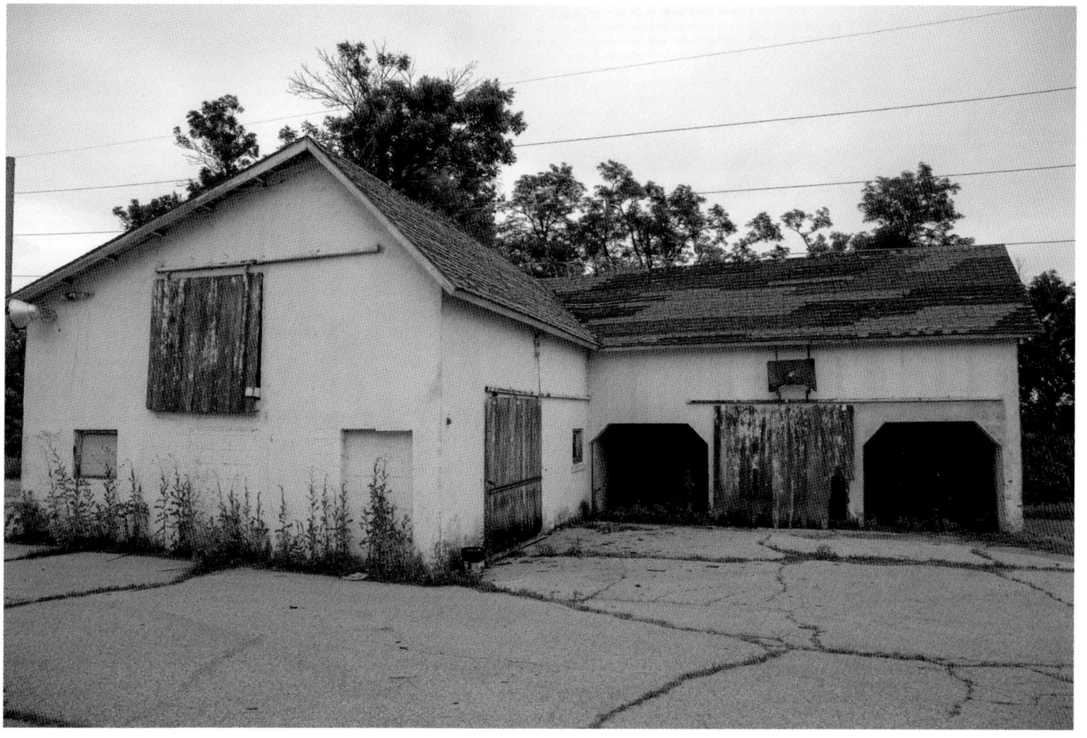

Garage building.

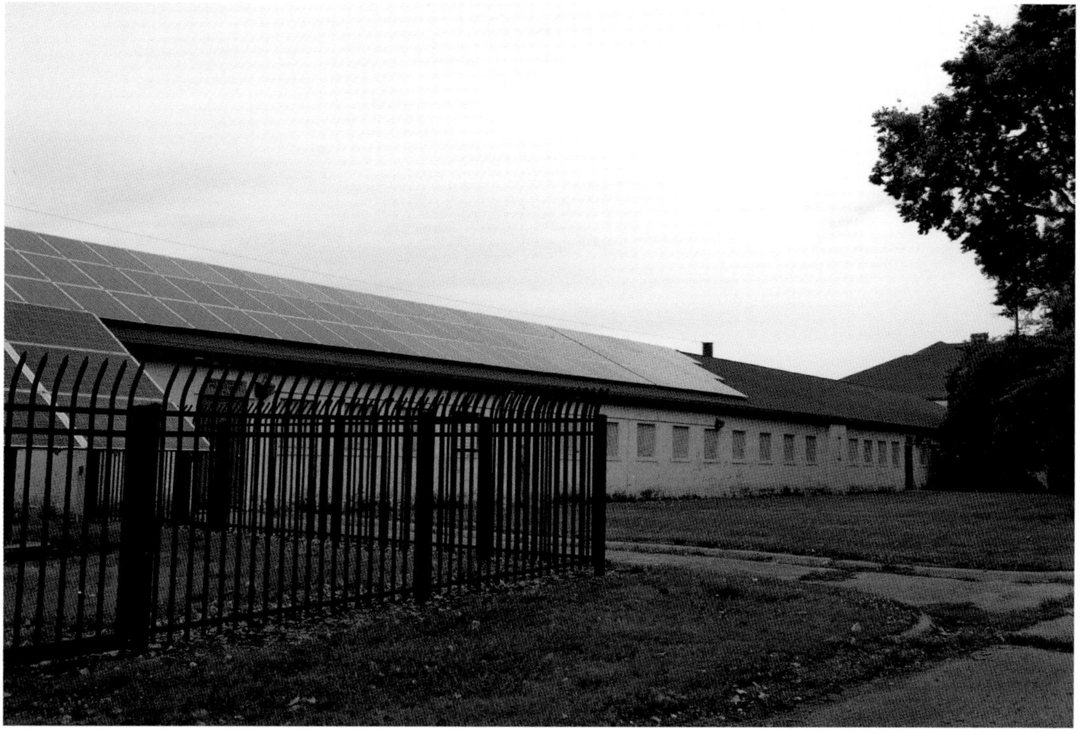

Evergy now utilizes the roof of the dairy barn for solar panels.

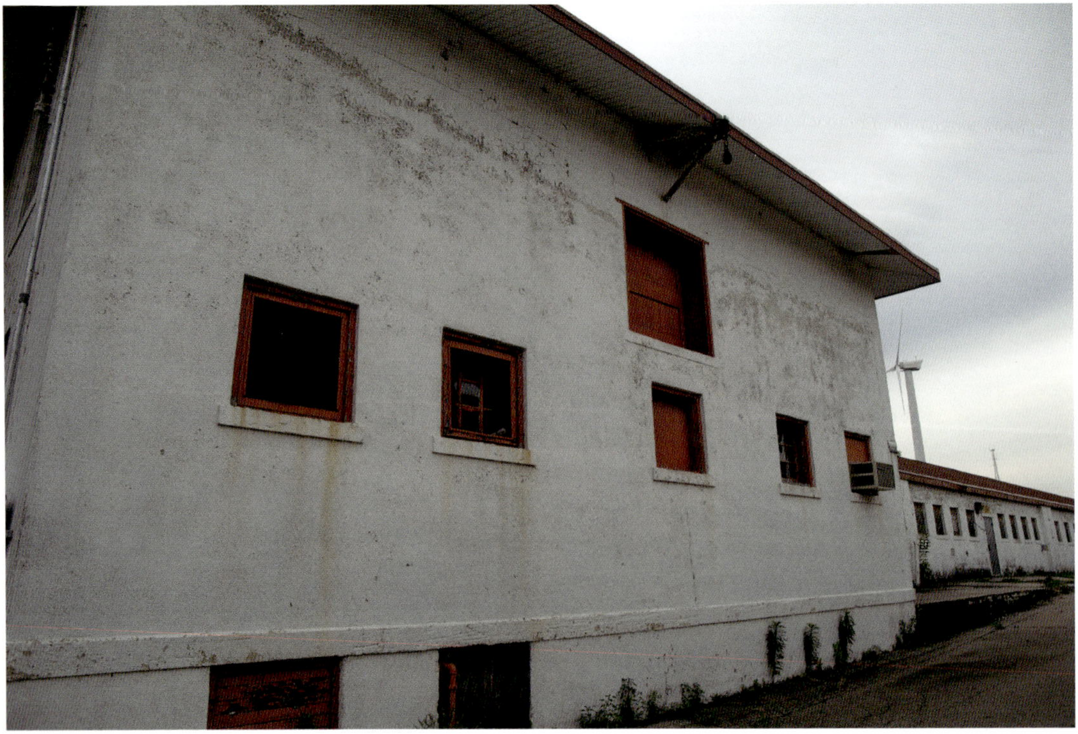

A pulley system sits above this window.

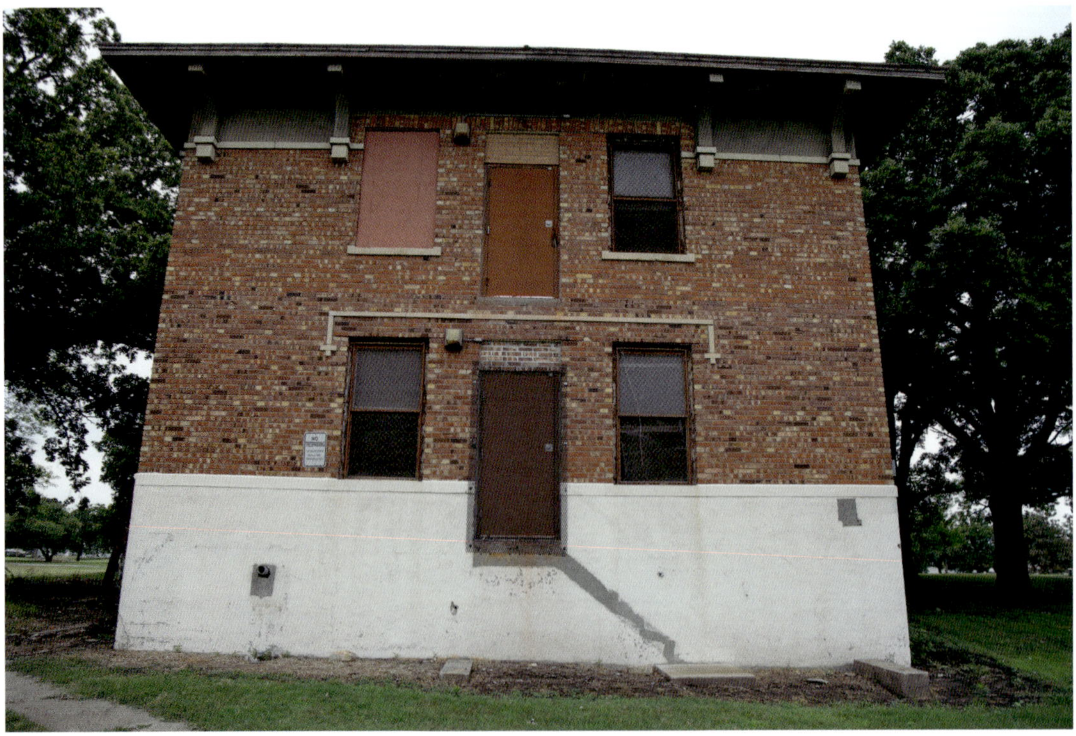

Stairway to nowhere.

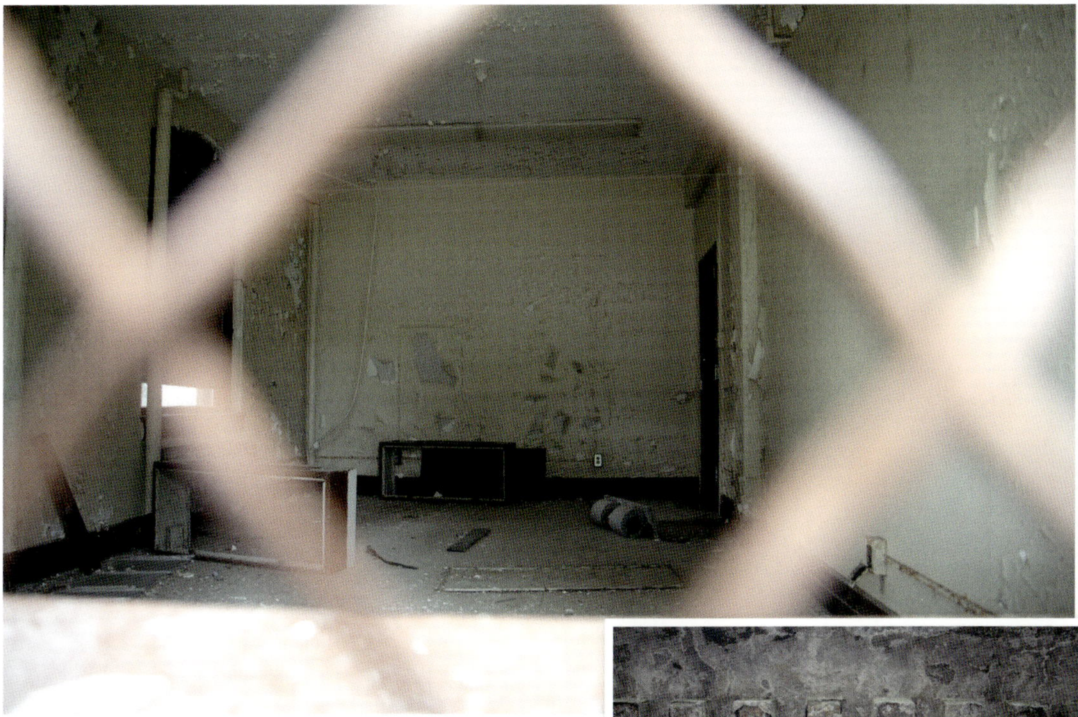

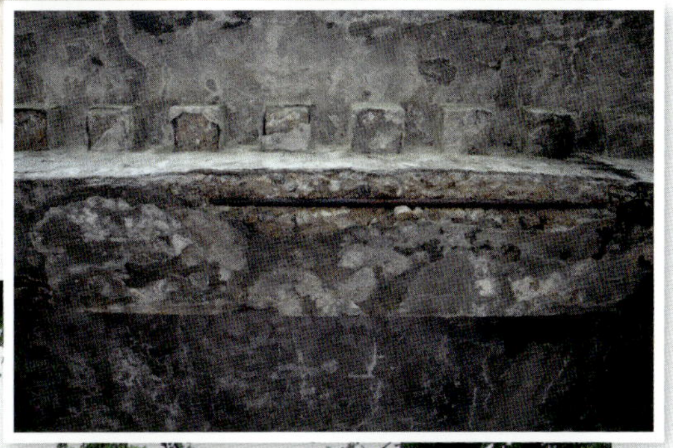

This building is in relatively good condition compared to the others. *Inset:* Textures of concrete.

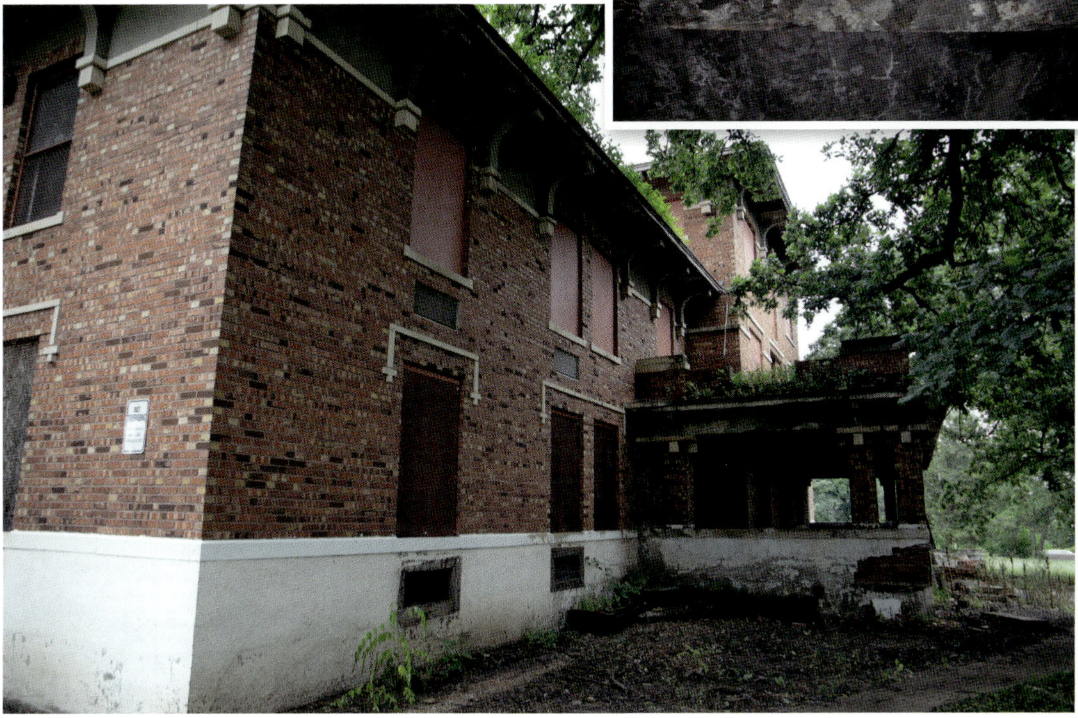

K Psychiatric Building.

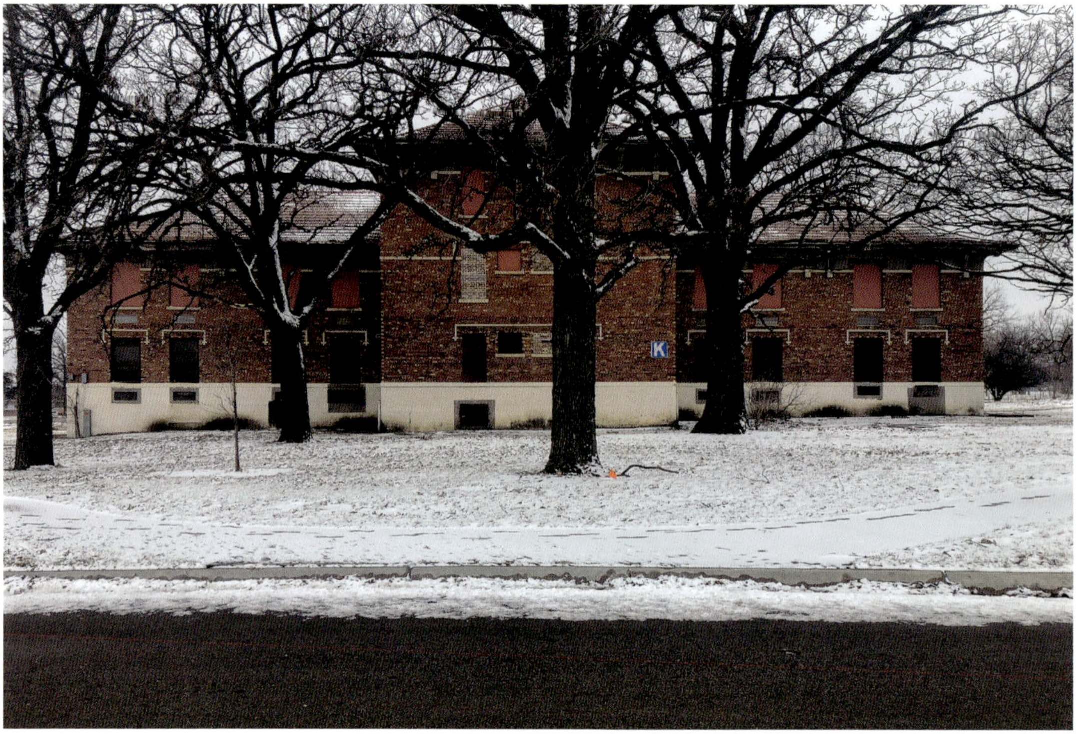

K Psychiatric Building.

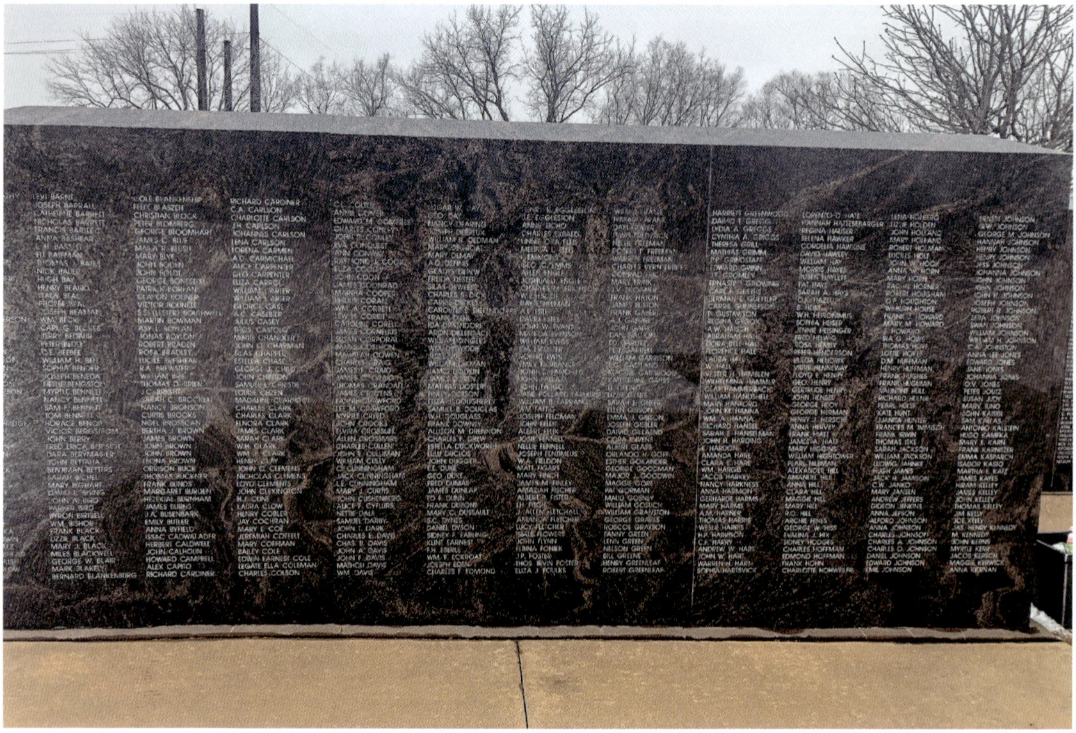

Memorial stone 1.

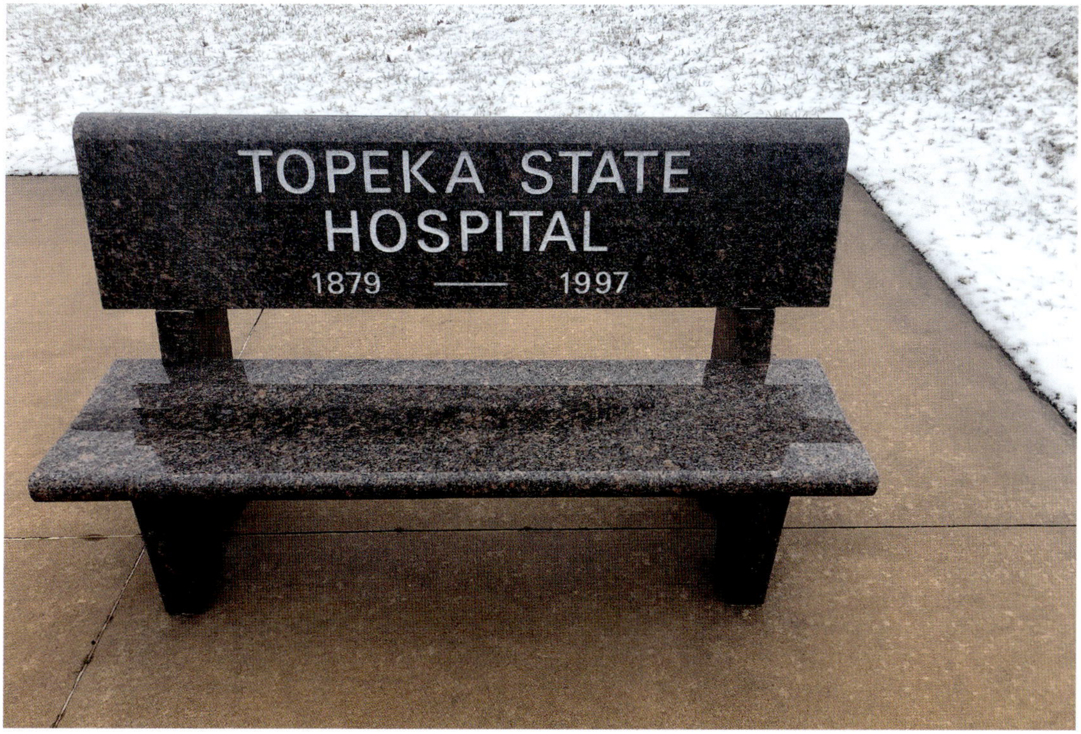

Memorial bench in the cemetery.

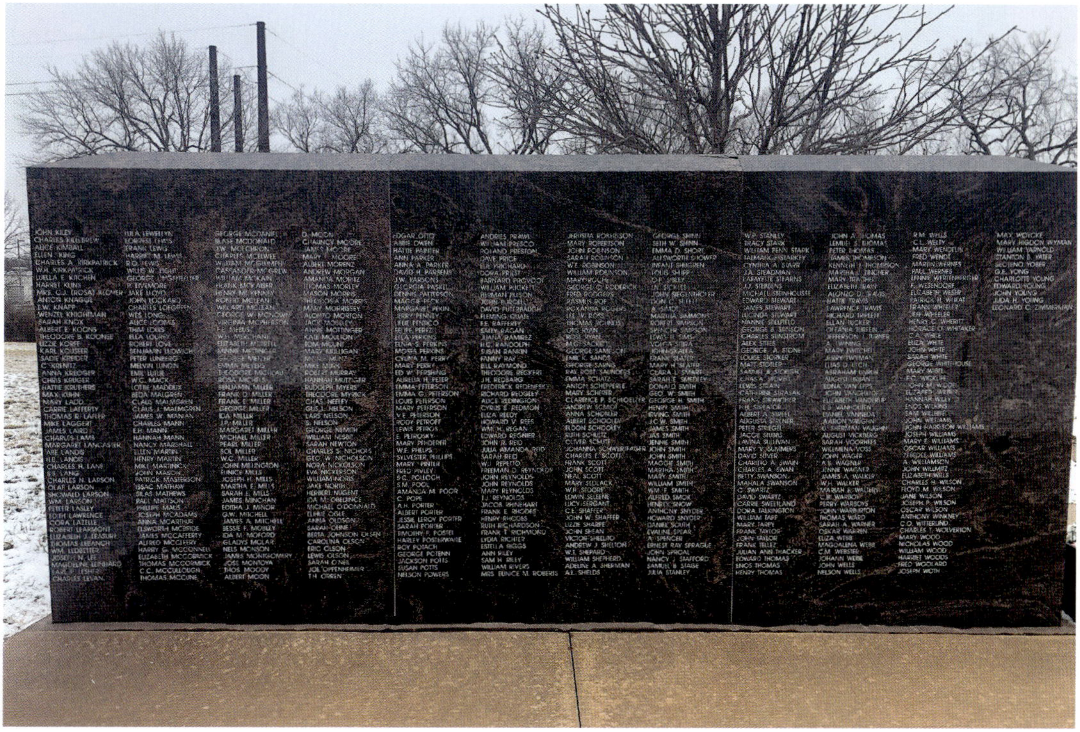

Memorial stone 2.

BIBLIOGRAPHY

"2 Contracts Let; Board Hears Kicks," *The Topeka Daily Capital* (Topeka: 1914), p. 8, Newspapers.com.

"Another School Case," *The Ottawa Daily Republic* (Ottawa: 1880), p. 4, Newspapers.com.

"Authorities Investigate Hotel Death," *St. Joseph Gazette* (St. Joseph: 1987), p. 24, Newspapers.com.

Blankenship, Bill. "East Topeka Junior High's Last Graduating Class Plan Reunion," *The Topeka Capital-Journal* (Topeka: 2016), Cjonline.com.

"Bond Election is Asked by Board of Education," *The Parsons Daily Sun* (Parsons: 1911), p. 1, Newspapers.com.

"Breakfast Table Chat," *The Topeka Daily Capital* (Topeka: 1919), pp. 8-10, Newspapers.com.

"Building Is Safe," *The Topeka Daily Capital* (Topeka: 1898), p. 5, Newspapers.com.

Chilson, Morgan "Former Red Carpet Inn Faces Uncertain Future," *The Topeka Capital-Journal* (Topeka: 2018), Cjonline.com.

"Construction," *Topeka This Week* (Topeka: 1926), p. 10, Newspapers.com.

"Editorials," *The Topeka Daily Capital* (Topeka: 1915), p. 8, Newspapers.com.

"Enlarge McKinley School," *The Topeka Daily Capital* (Topeka: 1922), p. 6, Newspapers.com.

"Ex-school said now Unsafe for seniors but not Christian Academy," *The Manhattan Mercury* (Manhattan: 2005), p. 3, Newspapers.com.

"Famed Psychiatric Clinic Abandons Prairie Home," *The New York Times* (New York: 2003), p. 1, Nytimes.com.

"Former Students of Topeka's All Black Schools Share Their Stories," *WIBW News Channel 13* (Topeka: 2019), p. 1, Wibw.com.

"Glimpses at McKinley School," *The Topeka Daily Capital* (Topeka: 1919), p. 4, Newspapers.com.

Grossman, Ron. "Era Ends for Menningers," *Chicago Tribune* (Chicago: 2018), p. 1, Chicagotribune.com.

Handy, Pauline "Interviewed," *The Topeka Plaindealer* (Topeka: 1923), p. 3, Newspapers.com.

"History of McKinley School," *The Topeka Daily Capital* (Topeka: 1914), p. 8, Newspapers.com.

Hrenchir, Tim. "Foundation Renovates Historic Menninger Buildings," *The Topeka Capital-Journal* (Topeka: 2019), p. 1, Cjonline.com.

"Image 23 of Sanborn Fire Insurance Map from Topeka, Shawnee County, Kansas." *The Library of Congress*, www.loc.gov.

"In City Schools," *The Topeka Daily Herald* (Topeka: 1906), p. 9, Newspapers.com.

Jones, Corey. "Vacant Hotel Near Downtown Being Gutted," *The Topeka Capital-Journal* (Topeka: 2011), Cjonline.com.

Kidd, Tim "Racial Bias dying slow death years after school ruling," *Dayton Daily News* (Dayton: 1979), p. 15, Newspapers.com.

"MALL HALL OF FAME," mall-hall-of-fame.blogspot.com.

"Malls of America," Mallsofamerica.blogspot.com

"May Get City Water," *The Shawnee Chief* (Topeka: 1914), p. 1, Newspapers.com.

"Minor Incidents," *The Topeka State Journal* (Topeka: 1896), p. 2, Newspapers.com.

"Much School Business," *The Topeka State Journal* (Topeka: 1895), p. 8, Newspapers.com.

"National Register of Historic Places Registration Form," *NPGallery Search*, Npgallery.nps.gov/GetAsset/87ddda29-f120-416f-8ae0-178372224049.

"New Sumner School Building Will Be Brought into Use," *The Topeka Daily Herald* (Topeka: 1902), p. 6, Newspapers.com.

"NPGallery Asset Detail," npgallery.nps.gov/AssetDetail/NRIS/03001397.

"On School Risks," *The Topeka State Journal* (Topeka: 1910), p. 5, Newspapers.com.

Smith, Sherman, "St. Francis Deal Allowed Denver Nonprofit to Keep Menninger Hill, Cash, Artifacts," *The Topeka Capital-Journal* (Topeka: 2011), p. 1, Cjonline.com.

"Snap Shots at Home News," *The Topeka State Journal* (Topeka: 1922), p. 10, Newspapers.com.

"Snapshots," *The Topeka State Journal* (Topeka: 1908), p. 10, Newspapers.com.

"Statement of Fact About the Bonds," *The Parsons Daily Sun* (Parsons: 1911), p. 1, Newspapers.com.

"Students Are Pleased," *The Topeka Daily Capital* (Topeka: 1919), p. 10, Newspapers.com.

"Sumner School Repaired," *The Topeka State Journal* (Topeka: 1895), p. 3, Newspapers.com.

"Sumner School Will Soon Be Ready for Use," *The Topeka State Journal* (Topeka: 1902), p. 16, Newspapers.com.

"Sumner School," *The Daily Commonwealth* (Topeka: 1885), p. 4, Newspapers.com.

"Sumner School," *The Topeka Daily Press* (Topeka: 1894), p. 4, Newspapers.com.

"Sunflower Foundation," *Sunflower Foundation* (Topeka: 2020), Sunflowerfoundation.org.

"The Menninger Clinic, A Farmhouse in 1925, Now a World Center," *The New York Times* (New York: 1975), p. 1, Nytimes.com.

"To Sell Sumner School," *The Topeka State Journal* (Topeka: 1899), p. 4, Newspapers.com.

"Topeka's Educational Edifices," *The Topeka Daily Capital* (Topeka: 1880), p. 4, Newspapers.com.

"Foundation Has a Vision for Former Menninger Campus," *The Wichita Eagle* (Wichita: 2016), p. 3, Newspapers.com.

"Menninger Clinic Grounds to be State Park," *The Hays Daily News* (Hays: 2006), p. 8, Newspapers.com.

"Menninger's Archive Gets Topeka Home," *The Hays Daily News* (Hays: 2004), p. 37, Newspapers.com.

Milburn, John. "Demolition of Menninger Campus Begins," *Plainview Herald* (Plainview: 2016), p. 1, Myplainview.com

"Proposed Plan of Security Benefit Association in Topeka When Completed With 15 Buildings," *The Topeka State Journal* (Topeka: 1922), p. 12, Newspapers.com.

"Security Benefit Addition to be Built at Cost of $350,000," *The Frankfort Index* (Frankfort: 1928), p. 6, Newspapers.com.

"Security Benefit Association Now Thirty Years Old," *The Topeka Daily Capital* (Topeka: 1922), p. 28, Newspapers.com.

Wims-Campbell, Carolyn L. "Legacy of Brown: Education Leader Never Felt 'at Risk,'" *The Topeka Capital-Journal* (Topeka: 2014), p. 1, Cjonline.com.